THE HISTO
OF *NATURAL* H.

The Basic Teachings Of Doctors
Jennings, Graham, Trall & Tilden

By
Hereward Carrington, Ph. D.
Author of "Vitality, Fasting & Nutrition," "The Natural Food of Man,"
"Fasting for Health and Long Life," "Death Deferred," etc.

AND

Principles of Natural Hygiene

By
Herbert M. Shelton, N. D.

First Published in 1954

Martino Publishing
Mansfield Centre, CT
2010

Martino Publishing
P.O. Box 373,
Mansfield Centre, CT 06250 USA

www.martinopublishing.com

ISBN 1-57898-873-X

© *2010 Martino Publishing*

Cover design by T. Matarazzo

Printed in the United States of America On 100% Acid-Free Paper

THE HISTORY
OF *NATURAL* HYGIENE

The Basic Teachings Of Doctors
Jennings, Graham, Trall & Tilden

By
Hereward Carrington, Ph. D.
Author of "Vitality, Fasting & Nutrition," "The Natural Food of Man,"
"Fasting for Health and Long Life," "Death Deferred," etc.

AND

Principles of Natural Hygiene

By
Herbert M. Shelton, N. D.

First Published in 1954

HEALTH RESEARCH

California

DEDICATED TO

Isaac Jennings, M. D., Sylvester Graham, R. T. Trall, M. D., J. H. Tilden, M. D., and Herbert M. Shelton, N. D.

These five doctors had the mental capacity to think of a first principle in the art of healing. Their analysis of the basic cause of disease and the development of the components of a SYSTEM of natural methods of care and living has created the basic framework of *Natural Hygiene*.

TABLE OF CONTENTS

List of Illustrations

FOREWORD

The thoughtful student of any school of thought is always concerned with the origin of the views composing the group of ideas of his interest.

Recognizing this need, Hereward Carrington, Ph. D., brilliant writer and student of *Natural Hygiene* has carefully analyzed and selected the basic writings of those who have so painstakingly developed the principles of *Natural Hygiene*. These extractions are included in the text of this volume—in fact compose a large portion of it. The arrangement is such as to present the evolvement and growth of the basic ideas of the *Hygienic System*. For a short title we have chosen *The History of Natural Hygiene* (although the history of this great movement could never be given in such a small booklet).

It is interesting to note that three of the five contributors were Medical Doctors of standing in their time. These men after years of practice of Medicine in the approved and traditional form recognized its inadequacies and failures to meet the need of sick humanity—even as many of the Medical Doctors of today feel helpless in the face of repeated failures.

But these men had the courage to challenge the worn out tradition and theory of their professions and seek a new approach to man's age-old search for health. Their success in uncovering the basic principles of *Natural Hygiene* is a tribute to their perserverance and intelligence.

A study of the text which follows will not only provide the student with a historical sequence of the development of the ideas composing the *Hygienic System*, but will give a better understanding of these ideas as well.

R. G. WILBORN, D. C., N. D.,

THE BASIC HEALTH TEACHINGS OF ISAAC JENNINGS, M.D.

By Hereward Carrington

Dr. Isaac Jennings was a contemporary of Trall and Sylvester Graham, flourishing during the latter half of the last century; but his work is comparatively little known—being perhaps partially eclipsed by the scintillating brilliance of their writings, and partially by the relative moderation of his claims. Yet he was a great and sincere health-reformer, and it is unfortunate that his style of writing was so ponderous, and was interspersed throughout with religious and anecdotal material which seems somewhat boring to the average reader today.

Jennings called his own system of medication "Orthopathy," and he published a number of books, the chief being "Philosophy of Human Life," "Medical Reform," and "The Tree of Life." He was a close friend of William A. Alcott and for years associated with Prof. C. G. Finney, of Oberlin, Ohio, a famous adventist-theologian of his day. It is only natural, therefore, that his books should be theological in tone, for, like Graham, he was brought up in that atmosphere.

All this, however, does not detract from his writings on hygiene, since he was first and last a physician—but one who, after more than twenty years of inner struggle, saw "the light of day" and launched himself fervently into the crusade for health-reform, which was then at white heat. He violently attacked "doctors" and drug medication, and aroused the ire of his medical bretheren in consequence. To these attacks he replied at length.

Jennings had a quaint style of his own, but his basic teachings may perhaps be summarized as follows:

"The general law of the human economy is a unit. In all its operations, as a general rule, whether the result be perfect or impaired health, its tendency is one and indivisible; the highest and best interest of the whole system." For the purpose of showing its nature, tendency and adaptation to the purposes of life and health, this is examined under a number of Divisions. These are:

First: The Law of Action (Exercise).

Second: The Law of Repose (sleep, rest).

Third: The Law of Economy (to husband the vital energy).

Fourth: The Law of Distribution (supplying each part of the body with vital energy).

Fifth: The Law of Accomodation (adjustment to poisons, etc.

Sixth: The Law of Stimulation ("sounding the alarm" in danger).

Seventh: The Law of Limitation (prevention of the waste of vital energy by Nature).

Eighth: The Law of Equilibrium (re-vitalization of weak spots).

These Jennings thought the eight most vital laws of life.

Attempting to define "What Disease Is," Jennings says:

"Impaired health or disease is simply a lower degree of the action of parts affected, than is performed by the same parts in their highest state of health, together with such defects in the solids and fluids as flow from such depressed action. . . . When the tide of vital energy is on the full flood, the action of the organ will be at the highest point of health for any given condition of the organ. And as the tide of energy ebbs, the condition of the organ in other respects continuing the same, its action declines in the same ratio as long as a sufficient quantity remains to move it at all. . . . I affirm that *lack of vital energy* is the immediate, generic reason why derangements of any kind are suffered to take place in the human system. . . ."

This, it will be observed is virtually identical with the "enervation," stressed by Tilden, Shelton and others, as a basic factor in the genesis of "disease."

As *causes* of this depletion of the vital energies, Jennings mentions excessive exertion, dietetic errors, tea, coffee and alcohol, sexual excesses, insufficient rest and sleep, emotional strains and stresses, etc. Much the same list would probably be made today.

Jennings then deals at length with the various "symptoms" of disease (cough, catarrh, fever, pain, irritability, etc.) which to us hardly seem worth the space devoted to them. He then launches forth into his defense of Vegetarianism, enumerating the various arguments now so familiar to us, and pointing out that meat-eating and a craving for alcohol usually go together. Inasmuch as Jennings was a militant temperance advocate, one can perhaps excuse the lengthy tirade he launches against alcoholism.

The reason that meat-eating and drinking are so often associated is that meat is the most stimulating of all *solid* foods; and, since greater and greater stimulation is constantly called for, once this vicious circle is started, this can only be found in liquid form, *i.e.*, alcohol.

It is of interest to note that Jennings, while defending the use of milk in the diet, wrote strongly against the use of butter and cheese, contending that they are both, in some degree, "poisonous."

In his day, any form of medication that did not consist in the administration of powerful drugs and violent purgatives was known as the "let alone" treatment; and this plan Jennings strongly advocated. In fact, he seems to have been at first inclined towards the Homeopathic School, on this account—not because of the "medicines" they gave, but because they did less harm than the allopaths. However, he was finally led to believe that they did not achieve the same results as he did, with his bread pills. Hence, he was led to attack them, too.

While realizing that most so-called "diseases" are self-limited, that they consist of more than a set of symptoms, that they should not be thwarted, and above all, that they were not dangerous enemies or entities, which "attack" the patient from outside, nevertheless Jennings failed to realize the true basic cause of such conditions, in the sense that Trall did, when he defined them as "remedial actions." Their true *rationale*—as well as the seeming "action" of drugs—Trall was the first

to enunciate clearly. He also failed to employ the skilled "guidance"
which Trall employed. Nevertheless, of course, Jennings did an immense
amount of good in his day, by reason of his attacks upon the orthodox
systems then in vogue, and by his advocacy of the "let alone" plan.

In discussing the diet of patients, Jennings has this to say:

"Food has no more to do with the production of vitality than the
timber, planks, bolts and canvas for a ship have in supplying ship-
carpenters and sailors. In the mass of diseases, and most of the disorders that are termed febrile, the proper course of treatment to be
pursued is exceedingly plain and simple. So long as there is no call
for nutriment, a cup of cool water is all that is needed for the inner
man. A good nurse, however, who knows how to humor the whims of
the patient, will often find enough to do in caring for the outer man.
Indulgences should be granted freely, when they are not positively or
seriously injurious. The great object to be steadily aimed at in all cases
of sickness is to favor the renovating process which is in constant pro-
gression within. *Rest, quiet,* is the great remedy. Let there be no unnecessary expenditure of vital funds, either through mental exercise, or
any undue exercise of the bodily functions. When there is a disposition
to sleep, let it be indulged. And as there is no medicine to be given
by the hour, sleep may be protracted to any length, unless it is laborious;
then a slight jog, or a little change of position, or a swallow of water,
will start it in its regular train again." *(The Tree of Life, p. 187).*

In his day, therapeutic fasting and relatively unknown, and it is
highly probable that Jennings himself was one of the first to advocate
a fast of many days, on nothing but water,—yet his writings show that
he actually did. Fashing began to gain acceptance with the turn of the
present century. What delight many of these old-time health-reformers
would have displayed, had they lived to witness our modern methods of
hygienic treatment!

Nevertheless, Jennings, of course, advocated great modification and
restriction in the diet. Speaking of this, he says:

"The quantity of food to be taken by the sick should be regulated
on the general principle that has been laid down for the regulation of
exercise; according to the demands of the system, to be measured or
ascertained by the promptings of nature, and the effects of what is taken.
In the most difficult or critical parts of the renovating operation, when
all the forces that can be mustered and spared are needed for the removal of defects, and laying a foundation for rebuilding, the nutritive
processes will be wholly suspended, so long as sustenance can be furnished to the laboring organs from depositions in the different parts of
the body; it being less expensive and more advantageous to the economy
of life, to sustain her workmen with nutriment that has been already
assimilated or animalized, than to manufacture and furnish it with raw
material. But when this source of supply fails, there is no alternative
but to clothe the organs of nutrition with power and call for raw material, or "give up the ship," for they that work must eat. While, therefore, there is no call for food, no disposition manifested by the stomach

to receive and use it, it will be in vain to urge food upon the stomach. And when a faint, feeble call is made for food, care must be taken not to over-feed, for here, too, the danger is on the side of overdoing. . .

In cases of great debility, the common belief is that food must be taken for the purpose of communicating strength; but this is as great a mistake as the supposition that exercise strengthens. Food carries no vital power into the system with it, but requires much to convert it into organized texture and endow it with vitality. Any quantity therefore that is taken into the system, beyond the ability of the nutritive apparatus to animalize, will do more hurt than good. . . . It will answer no good purpose to employ excitants to appetite. If there is not power enough to create appetite, the case is a hopeless one. Provocations can neither create power, nor make an appetite without power. The common non-professional rule of giving food in cases of debility, "little and often," will answer very well as a common one, by striking out the word "often."

And again, in writing on "Clinical Diet," Jennings says:

"So long as persons are confined to their beds without appetite, there is very little to be done for them by way of feeding. It is of no advantage to urge food upon the stomach when there is no digestive power to work it up. If nutrient substances lie a few hours in the warm bath of the stomach without being sufficiently vitalized to protect them from the action of chemical affinity, they will be converted into acrimonious fluids and gasses, and be sources of mischief.

"There is never any danger of starvation so long as there are reserved forces sufficient to hold the citadel of life and start anew its mainsprings. For when sustenance becomes a prime necessity, the digestive apparatus will be clothed with power enough to work up some raw material, and a call made for it proportioned to the ability to use it. A few simple articles of diet, and very simply cooked, should be relied upon, until there is considerable digestive ability well established. . . ."

What, then, are we to think of the teachings of Dr. Jennings, in view of our present knowledge? As a very young child, I remember our old family physician saying to my mother: "There are only two fundamentals of good health—open bowels and a clear conscience!"

Modern Hygienists would hardly consider this adequate; yet how sensible it sounds when we consider that it was uttered at a time when pills and powders were the order of the day, and the treatment of the sick consisted of little else To us, it may sound primitive enough, but it was at least a beginning. The same may be said, it seems to me, of the writings of Jennings, and many of the old-time health reformers. Their work has been carried forward and amplified a thousand-fold; but this should not make us overlook or minimize the value of their early efforts at medical reform. For they suffered—and contributed—much. They helped to lay the foundations of modern Hygiene, and, as Jennings himself says, at the close of one of his books: "When people learn and practice the art of right living, physicians may go back to their farms and workshops!"

THE BASIC HEALTH TEACHINGS OF
DR. SYLVESTER GRAHAM

Few people today realize, in all probability, that "Graham bread"—so popular until a few years ago—was named after Dr. Sylvester Graham, one of the earliest of the 19th-Century health reformers or hygienists. Indeed, even his name is known to relatively few—though his teachings exerted an enormous influence during the last century. It is high time, therefore, that due credit should be paid to him and to his memory.

Sylvester Graham was born in 1794, in Boston, and was the youngest of 17 children. He was a delicate child, and at the age of sixteen was thought to have "contracted consumption." Indeed, this naturally frail constitution remained throughout life, and—as he himself points out —it was only his reformed diet and his hygienic mode of life which enabled him to remain in active health and alive as long as he did.

Not long after he was born his father died, and Sylvester's mother (who cared for him part of the time) possessed a melancholy and morbidly religious mind, which doubtless exerted an influence on the naturally sensitive child—influencing him, later on, to join the Presbyterian Church and become a preacher. In a way, however, it was fortunate that he did so, as he became interested, through this, in temperance reform, and this in turn led to the study of physiology and health generally which culminated in his ultimate emergence as a great hygienic reformer. It was during this earlier period that he wrote his little book on "Chastity," and began his interest in moral and social reform. He wrote articles for magazines and a booklet entitled *An Apology*, which was a reply to those critics who pointed to Sylvester's own frail constitution as a refutation of his teachings. Graham's reply to such criticisms was that, only these had kept him alive, and in fact he died at a relatively early age—on 6 September, 1851, in his 58th year. As one contemporary said of him: "His mind had always been too active for his feeble frame, and his spirit escaped from its mortal tenament, where it had been so long struggling to work-out the happiness of the human race."

Graham's great work was *The Science of Human Life*—an enormous volume of 650 closely-printed pages. This was published in 1843. In style, the book is prolix and somewhat ponderous, and is marred—from our present point-of-view—by his occasional religious moralizing (a hang-over of his earlier training) and by his faith in phrenology, which is now completely outmoded. However, these are relatively minor defects, and do not materially detract from the mass of invaluable data which he accumulated and expounded.

A brief summary of the contents of his great book will serve to indicate its general scope and character. This may well be followed by a few quotations, which will illustrate his theories and ideas in greater detail.

The first eight chapters are devoted mainly to anatomy and physiology, while the ninth and tenth deal with man's mental and moral powers. Chapter 11 considers the question: "How long can man live?" In Chapter 12 we come to the general rules of hygiene. The succeeding eleven chapters are devoted to the question of diet and food reform, and in these Graham elaborates his arguments in favor of vegetarianism, and even a fruitarian diet. He was, in fact, one of the first to show the scientific basis on which a frugivorous diet rests.

The subjects discussed in the remaining chapters cover such topics as regularity in eating, through mastication, hygienic cookery (with attacks on salt, condiments and spices, tea, coffee, alcohol, etc.), the physiology of hunger, the quantity of food necessary to sustain life, the dangers of excess, fasting, sleep, air, bathing, exercise, and a series of attacks on drugs and orthodox medication. Graham was emphatic in his contention that so-called "epidemic diseases" could invariably be avoided by those who adopted the reformed diet and way of life. This viewpoint is now, as we know, maintained by Dr. Herbert M. Shelton and by many modern health reformers.

It will be evident, from the above general summary, that Dr. Graham's book covered practically the entire field of hygienic reform and, considering the fact that it was written more than 100 years ago, constitutes a remarkable document and a veritable classic, which should certainly be in the library of every health enthusiast. (The only trouble is in finding a copy—since the book is out of print and exceedingly scarce!)

And now a few quotations from his book. Writing of the general following of mankind, in their attitude towards health, medicine and doctors generally, he says:

"While in health, mankind prodigally wastes the resources of their constitution, as if the energies of life were inexhaustible; and when, by the violence of these excesses, they have brought on acute or chronic disease, which interrupts their pursuits and destroys their comforts, they fly to the physician, not to learn from him by what violation of the laws of life and health they have drawn the evil upon themselves, and by what means they can in future avoid the same and similar difficulties, but, considering themselves as unfortunate beings, visited with afflictions which they have in no manner been concerned in causing, they require the exercise of the physician's skill in the application of remedies, by which their sufferings may be alleviated and their diseases removed. And in doing this, the more the practice of the physician conforms to the appetites of the patient, the greater is his popularity, and the more cheerfully and generously is he rewarded.

How true! He further says:

"It is therefore beyond all question true that in all countries where human aliment is abundant and easily procured, gluttony or excessive alimentation is decidedly the greatest source of disease and suffering and premature death to man! 'Excess in drinking,' said Hippocrates, more than two thousand years ago, 'is almost as bad as excess in eating;' and the statement has remained true from that day to the present. Intoxicating liquors and substances, with all their fatal energy to destroy, and all the tremendous evils they have done—and surely they are great, terribly great!—have still caused less disease and pain and untimely death in the human family than errors in the *quantity* and quality of food! A drunkard sometimes, though very rarely, reaches old age; a glutton never does. . . .

However correct the quality of our food may be, if we habitually over-eat, our whole nature is injured, and always in proportion to our excess. Indeed it is, as a general rule, strictly true that a correct quantity of a less wholesome aliment is better for man than an excessively small or an excessively large quantity of a less wholesome aliment. . . .

The quantity of our food should, within certain limits, be proportionate to the amount of our active exercise; yet the most athletic and active laboring man is constantly in danger of taking too much food. Indeed, it is unquestionably true that at least ninety-nine percent of the farmers and other laboring men in New England are prematurely worn out and broken down by over-eating. All that exceeds the proper supply of the bodily wants necessarily oppresses the organs, diminishes the muscular power, and serves to impair and wear down all the energies of the system.*

The question is not whether man is capable of subsisting on a very great variety of vegetable and animal substances, for he does possess the constitutional capacity of deriving nourishment from almost everything in the vegetable and animal kingdoms; but the question is, do the highest interests of the human constitution indispensably require that man should, as a general rule, subsist on both vegetable and animal food? It is not whether he *can*, but whether he *must*, subsist on such a mixed diet, in order to secure the highest and best good of which his nature is capable. . . .

It has been judiciously observed that, when all the circumstances of civic life are taken into consideration, citizens generally should be regarded as invalids, by those who lay down rules of diet; for, although they may not be actually diseased, yet the causes which continually conspire to make them so are so numerous and so powerful that they need to use the caution and the prudence of invalids in order to preserve the health which they possess. Let it be understood, however, that the caution and prudence here suggested do not mean that citizens should be always taking medicine, or trembling lest a free breath of air should blow upon them, nor always thinking about their health, but that they should carefully avoid those excesses and errors in their dietetic and other habits which are decidedly unfavorable to human health. . . .

*Compare Rabagliati (Air, Food and Exercises, p. 237):

"If one should whisper to himself — what about poverty, then? — the very poor also eat too much or too often? It seems to me that they do. The poor eat poor food too often and too much, and the rich eat rich food too often and too much, and they are both ill . . . The charwoman is made ill and has her life shortened, not by insufficiency of diet, nor yet by the hard work which she is always talking about, but by the five meals which she thinks it necessary to take in order to 'keep up her strength' so as to be able to do her work. Even the beggar's baby suffers in the same way . . ."

If man subsisted wholly on uncooked food, the undepraved integrity of his appetite would greatly serve to prevent his over-eating, and thus save him from the mischievious effects of one of the most destructive causes operating in civic life. For excessive alimentation is undoubtedly the cause of more disease and premature death in civilized man than anything else which affects his existence; and there is no other possible way by which the evil can be removed than by a stern simplicity of diet rigidly adhered to throughout life. . . .

Ordinarily, dietetic changes should take place gradually—not that there is really so much danger in changing suddenly from a worse to a better diet, as is generally supposed, but that the uncomfortable feelings which at first attend such sudden changes are such as are almost certain to drive most people back to their old habits. . . .

It is infinitely better to subsist upon a mixed diet of vegetables and animal food, under a good general regime, than to live wholly on vegetable food badly selected, viciously prepared, and eaten in inordinate quantities, while at the same time we live in violation of almost every other correct rule of health. . . .

Were the constitutional principles, upon which the renovating capacity of the vital economy depends, in themselves inexhaustible, then were these bodies of ours, even in the present state of being, capable of immortality; but this is not so. *The vital constitution itself wears out!* The ultimate powers of the living organs are, under the most favorable circumstances, gradually expended and finally exhausted. . . .

In relation to disease, and the true principles and means of cure, the most universal and lamentable ignorance prevails amongst mankind. Few, probably, ever attempt to define their own notions on the subject, but are content to go through life with the most vague and indistinct impressions. Yet if we were to take the actions of men as true expressions of their ideas, we should unhesitatingly say that human beings almost universally consider health and disease as things absolutely and entirely independent of their own voluntary conduct, and of their ability to control. They regard diseases as substances or things which enter into their bodies with so little connection with their own voluntary actions and habits that nothing which they can do can prevent disease, nor vary the time nor the violence of its attack; and, according to their education, they believe it to be the effect of chance or of fate, or a direct and special dispensation of some Overruling Power. The consequence is that they either submit to disease as an element of their irresistible destiny, or seek for remedies which will kill it, or expel it from their bodies, as a substance or thing independent of the condition and action of their organs.

This latter notion is probably the most prevalent. People generally consult their physicians as those who are skilled in prescribing remedies that will kill disease; and these remedies they expect to act either as an antidote to a poison, or in some other way, with little or no reference to the condition and action of their organs, and to their dietetic and other voluntary habits. Many indeed seem to think that their physicians can take disease out of them and put health into them, by the direct application of remedies, and that there is, in the remedies themselves, a health-giving potency which, of its own intrinsic virtue, directly and immediately imparts health to the body.

This erroneous notion, as a matter of course, leads people to place their dependence on the sovereign virtue of remedies, and consequently to undervalue the highest qualifications of the truly scientific physician. ... The result of all this error is that, in the first place, mankind do not believe that their own dietetic and other voluntary habits and actions have much, if anything, to do with the preservation of health; and in the second place, when diseased, they expect to be cured by the sovereign power of medicine alone, and do not believe that any particular diet can of itself be of any great importance either in preventing or promoting their restoration to health. ...

All over-working, over-excitement, and irritation of the stomach and other organs concerned in the general function of nutrition necessarily cause an abatement of the sensorial power of the nervous system. And by over-working I do not mean merely that oppression of the stomach and other organs which is attended with immediate distress or uneasiness; but I mean all that exceeds the real wants of the vital economy, and is attended with a greater expenditure of vital power than is necessary to the healthy and perfect operations and results of the economy. Before the constitution has been broken down, while its springs are yet elastic and its energies are great, the most vigorous and high-toned health of body may be maintained for a considerable time without any of those painful feelings which tell us that we are excessively over-working the system, and warn us that we are pushing our health to the extremes which approach the very verge of violent disease and sudden death....

Indeed, it seems as if the grand experiment of mankind has ever been to ascertain how far they can transgress the laws of life, how near they can approach to the very point of death, and yet not die—at least so suddenly and violently as to be compelled to know that they have destroyed themselves. ... "

With the universal opinion, that all their diseases and sufferings were the direct and arbitrary and even vindicative inflictions of their God, or Gods, mankind have cherished no other fear of disease than that which grows out of their gross superstition—a fear that God would send sickness and death upon them, independently of any laws which He has established in relation to health and disease. *** It has never occurred to them that there is any relation between their own voluntary habits, customs, and indulgencies, and the diseases with which they are afflicted. *** They have never sought to find the causes of their diseases within the precincts of voluntary conduct; and have never taken any care to prevent disease, by avoiding its causes. The whole drift *** has been to this one point, on this subject—the ascertainment of *remedies* for disease in every form. And hence the phenomena or symptoms of disease have been studied *** less for the purpose of ascertaining the nature of the disease in re-

— 13 —

lation to its causes, than for the purpose of ascertaining what *remedies* are to be used. How could it be otherwise, amid such errors, than that disease should soon and universally come to be considered as a thing distinct from its causes, and consequently be treated with little or no reference to its causes—nay, indeed! the active causes be permitted to operate unsuspected; and yet worse, the causes be associated with the remedial agents; and worst of all, the very causes, themselves, be administered as remedial agents in the case. Such a delusion necessarily has led to the deeper and more fatal error, that there is in *medicine* an *intrinsic* health-giving virtue; that it has the power absolutely to take away or kill disease and impart health! And this has led the way to that wide-sweeping evil that has spread more calamitously than all the plagues of Egypt, over the whole *civilized* world; —the eternal and suicidal drugging! drugging! drugging! of mankind. Regarding disease as a thing apart from its causes; and believing medicine to possess an intrinsic, salutary potency; they have ignorantly and eagerly gathered upon themselves the causes of disease, and sought a redemption from the painful consequences only in the virtues of medicine, which has too often proved more destructive than the original causes themselves, and in co-operation with these causes, has terribly accelerated the work of death.

— SYLVESTER GRAHAM *in Esculapian Tablets,* 1837.

These sample extracts from Sylvester Graham's book will serve to give the reader an idea of his general philosophy and health teachings —which were original, daring and far in advance of his times. Much that he said has of course been amplified and brought up-to-date by modern authors, but credit must always be given them for their historical value—and to Dr. Graham himself for the profound and beneficial influence he exerted, not only in his own day, but for all time to come.

Well might we say of him: "The King is dead; long live the king!"

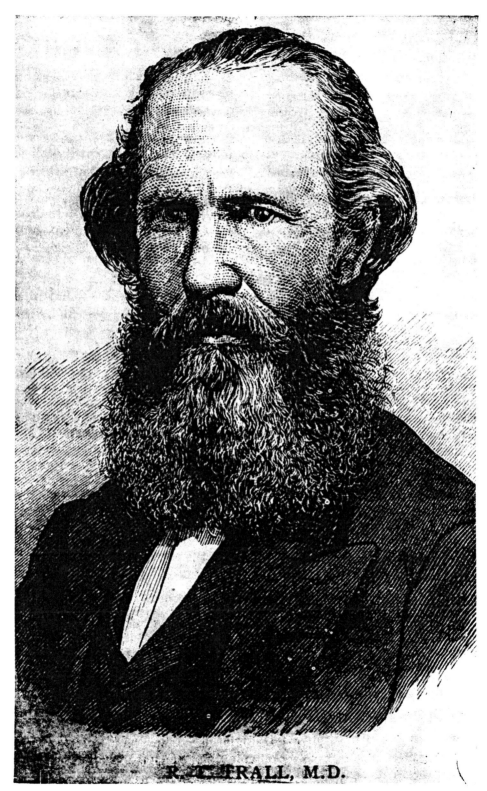

R. T. TRALL, M.D.

THE BASIC HEALTH TEACHINGS OF R. T. TRALL, M.D.

It is not too much to say that Dr. R. T. Trall was largely responsible for revolutionizing modern medicine and formulating the principles of natural hygiene. For, although many others had written before him —particularly Sylvester Graham—it was Trall who unified all this material, and consolidated it into a philosophical whole. It was he who employed all that was best in the old water-cure, in reformed diet, in exercise, in hygienic cooking, in the natural treatment of so-called diseases, who defended the scientific basis of vegetarianism, who pointed out the true "action" of drugs and alcoholic stimulants, but who, above all, showed the true nature of "disease," emphasizing the fact that all so-called diseases are in reality remedial efforts on the part of Nature, and as such cannot be "cured!" For all of which his name should go down in history as perhaps the greatest and most original of all health reformers.

Trall flourished about a hundred years ago; and in his time, drugging was the order of the day. The average physician thought of no other form of treatment, and the public had grown so used to the idea that health could be "bought in a bottle," that it never occurred to them that any other form of treatment was possible. Symptoms of a so-called "disease" were treated as the disease itself; and the main object of treatment was to smother and reduce these symptoms. Against this idea Trall protested strongly. He insisted that practically all diseases were in reality processes of cure—efforts on the part of nature to right a wrong; and went so far as to say that anyone who understands the mechanism of a sneeze should understand the nature of such diseases. For, just as foreign matter is violently expelled, in the process of sneezing, so is waste and morbid matter expelled by the body, in a set of symptoms noted by us, in the many so-called "diseases." Basically the process is the same. And, just as it would be absurd to try and smother the sneeze, so it is absurd to try and suppress the symptoms, which constitute the outward and visible signs of the curing processes going on in the body. We should aid and abet them, not hinder and prevent them. Disease itself is the process of cure. That was the basic element of his teaching.

Today we know that this is correct, and every advance in natural hygiene has emphasized this truth more and more fully. But in his day it was such a revolutionary idea that it met with violent opposition on all sides—and particularly, of course, by the orthodox medical profession —as indeed it does today!

Assuming its truth, however, what were the measures which Trall advocated to restore the sick person to health? Not by smothering symptoms, but by removing the *cause* of these symptoms—when they themselves would naturally and automatically disappear. What is this cause? Waste, poisonous material in the system, which nature is endeavoring to expel. Today this condition is known among health reformers as *toxemia*. By this they do not mean germs, or the excretions of germs, but a general condition of poisoning, brought on by an excess of putrefying waste material in the blood stream and body generally. When this is expelled, all symptoms (that is, all so-called diseases) spontaneously vanish. The patient is "cured."

The philosophy underlying "the true art of healing" is thus very simple. All so-called diseases are basically *one;* there are not many (local) diseases, but one causal factor, which may produce local symptoms. The same cause is at work, and the same methods of treatment are applicable in practically all cases.

As Trall said, in his "Hydropathic Encyclopedia," (Vol. II, p. 64): "All morbid actions are evidences of the remedial efforts of nature to overcome morbid conditions or expel morbid materials. All that any truly philosophical system of medication can do, or should attempt to do, is to place the organism under the best possible circumstances for the favorable operation of those efforts. We may thwart, embarrass, interrupt, or suppress them, as is usually the case, with allopathic practice, or we may direct, modify, intensify, and accelerate them, as is the legitimate province of hydropathic practice. But we must confess to the paradoxical proposition that the symptoms of disease are the evidences of the restorative effort; the effort, however, may be unequal to the end in view, and hence the powers of nature are to be assisted in removing obstacles, diverting irritation, etc."

This "morbid material" has accumulated within the system as the result, mainly, of our dietetic transgressions. We eat the wrong kind of food, and too much of it. Therefore, Trall advocated a rigid and abstemious diet, vegetarianism, properly combined foods, hygienic cookery, etc. He was also one of those who advocated fasting — which found its main champion, years later, in Dr. E. H. Dewey. Others had written in a general way on the value of this method of treatment; but few had ever applied it therapeutically, and in any systematic manner. Trall was one of the pioneers in this direction.

Writing on "the scientific basis of vegetarianism," Trall has this to say:

"Medical men teach us that animal food is stimulating. Here, for once, the premise is true. But stimulation and nutrition happen to be antagonistic ideas. Just so far as a thing stimulates, it does not nourish. Just so far as it nourishes, it does not stimulate.

"There is no more widespread delusion on earth than this, which confounds stimulation and nutrition. This is the parent source of that awful error — or rather, multitude of errors — which are leading all the nations of the earth into all manner of riotous living, and urging them on in the road to swift destruction. This terrible mistake is the prime cause of all the gluttony, all the drunkenness, all the dissipation, all the debauchery in the world — I had almost said, of all the vice and crime, also.

"But what is this stimulus of animal food? Let us see if we cannot understand it. What is a stimulant? It is anything which the vital

— 17 —

powers resist with violence and expel with energy. The disturbance of the organism which denotes the resistance, constituting a kind of feverishness, is stimulation. It is a morbid process. It is disease, hence a wasting process. Medical books have a class of medicines which are called stimulants. They are all poisons, and not foods. Anything which is foreign to the organism may provoke vital resistance, and in this sense be called a stimulant.

"But how does animal food stimulate? It always contains more or less effete materials—the debris of the disintegrated tissues, the ashes of the decayed organism—with more or less of other excrementitious matters. These impurities cannot be used in the organism, and therefore must be expelled; and this expulsive process, amounting to a feverish disturbance—this vital resistance—is precisely the rationale of the stimulating effects of animal food. And thus we prove that animal food is impure precisely in the ratio that it is stimulating, and for this reason objectionable.

"All that can be alleged in favor of flesh-eating, because of its stimulating properties, can be urged, and for precisely the same reasons, in favor of brandy-drinking or arsenic-eating."

Trall emphasizes here, indirectly, the true nature of alcoholic stimulation. Elaborating this idea in his "Alcoholic Controversy," he says: "We see how it is that alcohol is an element of force . . . It *occasions* force to be wasted. that is all. The system expends its force to get rid of the alcohol, but never *derives* any force, great or small, good, bad or indifferent, *from* the alcohol. Stimulation does not impart strength; it wastes it. Vital power does not go out of the brandy into the patient, but occasions vital power to be exhausted from the patient in expelling the brandy."

This also gives us the Key to the true "action" of drugs, which is, today, so much misunderstood. The mystery is clearly explained in the following passage from his pamphlet, "Water Cure for the Million":

"It is further taught, in all the books and schools of the drug-systems, that medicines have specific relations to the various parts, organs or structures of the living system; that they possess an inherent power to 'elect' or 'select' the part or organ on which to make an impression; and that, in virtue of this special 'elective' or 'selective' affinity, certain medicines act on the stomach, others on the bowels, others on the liver, others on the brain, others on the skin, others on the kidneys, etc. This absurd notion is the groundwork of the classification of the *materia medica* into emetics, cathartics, narcotics, diaphoretics, diuretics, etc. Now, the truth is exactly the contrary. So far from there being any such ability on the part of the dead, inert drug—any 'special affinity' between a poison and a living tissue—the relation between them is one of absolute and eternal antagonism. *The drugs do not act at all.* All the action is on the part of the living organism. And it ejects, rejects, casts out, expels, as best it can, by vomiting, purging, sweating, diuresis, etc., these drug poisons; and the doctors have mistaken this warfare *against* their medicines for their action on the living system."

Any drug, therefore, merely provokes a violent reaction on the part of the organism against it; and this reaction has been mistaken for action—the action of the drug! But it is always the living organism which acts. Give a purgative to a dead man, and there is no result. This only occurs when there is *life*. All that drugs can do is to waste energy and suppress symptoms. Their beneficial results are *nil*. They may occasionally relieve pain, but pain is a warning, on the part of nature, that something is wrong, calling for treatment. There is never pain without a cause. Remove the cause, and the pain will vanish. To subdue this pain without removing the cause is worse than useless. It is almost criminal. And yet it is upon this premise that much of modern "medicine" is founded—and the drug stores flourish! Surely, humanity badly needs to be educated in the principles of natural hygiene!

Trall also insisted upon the necessity for exercise, being one of the first to emphasize the truth that it is better for a man to 'wear out than to 'rust out.' Later researches on lymph circulation and the connective tissues have only emphasized this necessity. Few people realize that they have more lymph than blood in their bodies — only there is no heart to pump it, so that it moves slowly, unless stimulated by exercise Lymph congestion and the blockage of the connective tissues are both being recognized as important factors in the causation of so-called "diseases."

Trall also employed the "water cure" to a large extent, being careful, however, to weed-out its weaknesses and excesses. He was opposed to the *cold* water cure, contending that the temperature of the water should be gauged by the temperature of the patient's skin. If this was hot and feverish, then cold water was indicated. If, on the other hand, this was chilled, then hot packs, compresses and baths were in order.

When Dr. Trall entered the class room, there was one question he always asked first; and the class, knowing the answer, would call it out in unison. The question was: "When you are called to the bedside of a sick patient, what is the first thing to do?" And the class would respond: "Balance the circulation!" Usually, the internal organs, in any illness, are feverish and congested, while the skin is inactive. Therefore, draw the blood to the skin, and away from the inner organs. This could best be done by means of packs and compresses. Immediate relief is thus effected — and other treatment can then be commenced.

While Dr. Trall was a great believer in action, in activity, he also appreciated the necessity for sleep and rest. He often remarked that "a life cannot be both *in*tensive and *ex*tensive." If the vital energies are expended lavishly, then trouble is bound to follow; at the same time, a life devoid of activity is sure to reduce the energy-level at which one lives. A man cannot claim to be well merely because he is not obviously sick; he should live on a *high level* of vitality.

This can best be assured by moderation and living a truly hygienic life.

The importance of the right combinations of foods, and their proper cooking, were emphasized at length by Dr. Trall. He devoted a goodly share of his "Hydropathic Encyclopedia" to these questions, and wrote, in addition, his "Hygienic Home Cook Book." Much has been learned since his day on these topics, but the basic principles he enunciated are nevertheless as true now as ever.

The following extracts, culled here and there from Trall's writings, will illustrate at once the clarity and vision of his teachings, and the philosophy underlying them. Thus, in answer to various hypothetical questions, he says:

What is health?

Health is normal vital action — "the normal play of all the functions"; and this means that state or condition in which each organ and part performs its own proper duty.

What is disease?

Disease is just the opposite — abnormal vital action; and this means a state or condition of unbalanced circulation, in which some organs and parts do more and others less than their own appropriate work.

What are the conditions of health?

The proper use of those materials which are normally related to the living organism, and which are usually termed Hygienic agencies; coupled with the negative condition, the abuse or misuse of nothing.

What are the causes of disease?

They are innumerable; but for all practical purposes they may all be resolved into the misuse or abuse of Hygienic agencies, the introduction of poisons into the system, and the retention of waste or effete matters which constitute the impurities of the system. . . .

Practically, all diseases may be regarded and treated as conditions of obstruction, modified and complicated according to the existing causes.

What universal rule for medication does this imply?

It implies the leading indication that exists in all possible forms of disease; namely, to balance the circulation and temperature, and supply such conditions as will enable the organs to remove the obstructive matter, and recover the normal condition. . . .

The danger in all diseases consists in the morbid action being directed to, or concentrated in, one organ or part, instead of being distributed through many or all. Keeping the body, therefore, of an equal temperature all over the surface, by means of warm or cool applications, according to circumstances, tends to equalize functional duty.

How do food and poisons differ?

Poisons are non-usable things, which the living system is obliged to resist and expel. Everything, therefore, which is taken into the system and cannot be used, is a cause of disease, and the vital powers are obliged to expend more or less of their energies in getting rid of it. This is why poisons in small quantities occasion debility, and in large quantities, death.

What is the rule for drinking water?

According to thirst. It is better to drink little or nothing at meals. If the food is plain and unseasoned, eating does not produce thirst. . . .

In other places, Trall goes on to say:

It is also taught, in all of their books and schools, that disease is an entity, a thing foreign to the living organism, and an enemy to the life-principle. The truth is exactly the contrary. Disease is the life-principle at war with an enemy. It is the defender and protector of the living organism. It is a process of purification. It is an effort to remove foreign and offensive materials from the system, and to repair the damages the vital machinery has sustained. It is a remedial effort. Disease, therefore, is not a foe to be subdued, or "cured" or killed; but a friendly office to be directed and regulated. And every attempt to cure or subdue disease with drug-poisons, is nothing more nor less than a war on the human constitution. . . .

And, in answering one of his critics who said, "persons who live according to your system until they get well, are obliged to continue the system, or they are liable to get sick again," Trall replied: "And so they should be! A reformed drunkard can remain sober no longer than he lets intoxicating drink alone. Our system does not propose to avoid the penalties or disobedience to nature's laws. It is predicated on obedience to them. . . ."

Despite the seriousness of his writings, Trall himself had a keen sense of humor. Thus, in his "True Temperance Platform," (p. 45) he says: "A very pretty sum for cyphering would be: If one gallon of alcohol will *kill* a whale, one quart *destroy* a horse, one gill *finish* a turtle, one drachm *paralyze* a frog, one scruple *dement* a sparrow, and one drop *extinguish* a shrimp, how much will be required to *vitalize* an infant, *restore* a child, *strengthen* a youth, or *cure* an adult?"

And again, in his "Scientific Basis of Vegetarianism," he says: "They say that vegetable food is not sufficiently nutritious. But chemistry proves the contrary. So does physiology. So does experience. Indeed, it can be demonstrated that many kinds of fruit are nearly as nutritious as flesh. Many kinds of vegetables are quite as much so, and the grains and nuts several times as nutritious. They allege that human beings cannot have permanent strength without the use of animal food, right in face of the fact that the hardest work is now being done, and has always been done, by those who use the least animal food; and right in face of the fact, too, that no flesh eating animals can endure prolonged and severe labor. I should like to see them try the experiment of working a lion or a tiger, or a hyena, against an ox, a camel or a mule. Examples exist here and there, all over the world, of men of extraordinary powers of endurance who do not use animal food at all; and history is full of such examples in all ages of the world. And again: the largest and strongest animals in the world are those which eat no flesh-food of any kind—the elephant and rhinoscerous."

Dr. Trall himself was a prodigious worker. In addition to his extensive practice, he carried on for many years health-cure establishments, and edited a magazine. He also wrote articles and delivered lectures. His books, however, constitute his most important legacy to us, and a collection of these should be in the library of every true health reformer. (I have a complete set of these myself, and would not part with them for love or money.) Inasmuch as many today are relatively unfamiliar with his work, the following list may prove of value — the title of the book being followed by the year of publication:

Hydropathic Encyclopedia (2 vols.)	1851
Hydropathic Cook Book	1853
Uterine Disease and Displacements	1854
The Alcoholic Controversy	1855
The Family Gymnasium	1857
Sexual Abuses	1858
Water Cure for the Million	1860
Scientific Basis of Vegetarianism	1860
Diseases of the Throat and Lungs	1860
Diphtheria	1862
The True Healing Art	1862
The True Temperance Platform	1862
Sexual Physiology and Hygiene	1866
Hygienic Handbook	1872
Digestion and Dyspepsia	1873
Mother's Hygienic Handbook	1874
Hygeian Cook Book	1874
Popular Physiology	1875
Health Catechism	1875
The Human Voice	1875

His projected work, "The Principles of Hygienic Medication" never saw the light of day, being prevented by his untimely death. This was brought about partly by persistent over-work and partly by neglect. Dr. Trall was so busy with the affairs of others that he gave little thought to himself. He constantly drove himself, sometimes far into the night. He lived quite alone, but of course no one ever thought that anything could possibly happen to the great Dr. Trall. But "all men are mortal," and he was no exception to the rule!

But, though Dr. Trall is gone, his philosophy and his writings still remain, and today they constitute an invaluable groundwork of knowledge for every true health reformer. May his name long be remembered by hygienists everywhere! One day, doubtless, he will receive the homage and gratitude of mankind, which has been too long neglected. He was perhaps the greatest medical reformer of all time.

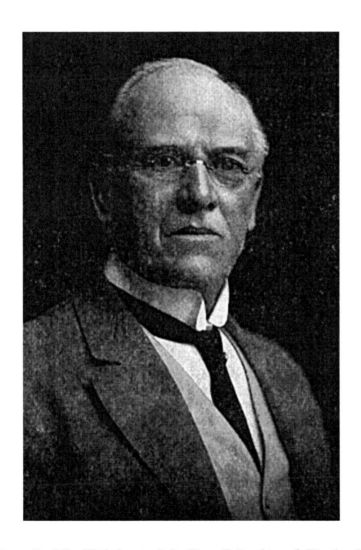

Dr. J. H. Tilden, M. D. (Medical Rebel)

THE BASIC HEALTH TEACHINGS OF DR. J. H. TILDEN

For hundreds and hundreds of years, "medical science" has maintained more or less the same viewpoint, and has made almost no progress! Compared with the other sciences it has remained static. True, some writer here and there had raised a voice of protest — even among the ancients; but their protests had been overlooked or forgotten, and had made no real impression upon the world as a whole, or the medical profession generally. Disease was still looked upon as an entity, something objective which could be "caught," or remained mysterious and inexplicable. Fads and "cures" of all kinds had arisen, only to be discarded by the next generation. Drugging had increased by leaps and bounds, and, later, the germ-theory was seized upon and accepted as the origin of many so-called "diseases." But, through it all, the same fundamental error remained — that innumerable separate and "local" diseases existed, which must be "cured" by the administration of drugs. And when the symptoms subsided, the disease was supposed to have been cured! Diseases and symptoms were so inter-locked, in the minds of medical men, that they were regarded as virtually synonymous. The effects were treated as the cause — and no one stopped to inquire what that cause was.

Even today this same viewpoint exists, and practically the whole of "modern medicine' is based upon this false viewpoint. Is it any wonder that little or no progress was made towards a rational system of treatment, so long as this primary error was accepted? It was only when this major premise was shown to be erroneous that light began to glow in the prevailing darkness, and a true philosophy of health could be formulated. This came about within the last century — almost within our own generation. What strides have been made since then!

Two men, above all others, must be given the credit for this initial reform. They were Sylvester Graham and R. T. Trall. Their basic teachings are no doubt familiar to my readers, and have been summarized elsewhere. Briefly, they were there: All so-called diseases, so far from being malign entities, are remedial efforts on the part of nature to right a wrong — curative processes which are noted in a set of symptoms. As such they cannot, of course, be "cured." They are themselves the indications of the cure. Practically all "diseases" are basically one — due to the same cause, and subject to the same mode of treatment. To reduce or smother these symptoms is not to "cure the disease," since its cause has not been eradicated. This cause is, in virtually all cases, morbid, poisonous material which is blocking the system and preventing its healthy functioning. When this cause is removed, health is restored. In this, drugs are useless; worse, they are positively harmful. Cleanse the system of this morbid material and health is automatically restored. Helping nature to do so is the only "treatment" required. Nature alone cures; all that we can do is to aid and assist her in her efforts. This can best be accomplished by simple, hygienic methods. There are no local, separate diseases, but local manifestations of a general condition. Remove the casual factor, and all "diseases" will automatically disappear.

The most we can do is to help nature in effecting this result. Normal health will then be restored.

Now, it will be observed that these ideas are diametrically opposed to those generally maintained — that disease must be fought and combatted, like some evil spirit which has entered the body of the patient. Instead they are beneficient and helpful! No wonder they aroused violent opposition when first promulgated!

These teachings of Trall's laid the foundations for the "nature cure" systems which subsequently developed. The Water Cure of Seb. Kneipp was welcomed, as well as the reformed diet, now well under way. Other hygienic measures were added, and found exponents in the persons of Felix Oswald, Charles E. Page, Aug. Reinhold, and many others — while the teachings of Dr. Edward Hooker Dewey, on fasting, were welcomed as of fundamental importance. At the beginning of this century these teachings found two powerful propagandists—Bernarr Macfadden and Dr. J. H. Tilden. The former launched his magazine "Physical Culture" in March, 1899; and the first issue of "The Stuffed Club" appeared in May, 1900. Both of these magazines exerted an enormous influence over the general public, and they were followed by a number of books by these same authors. Since then, hundreds of works have appeared, spreading these teachings, until today, as we know, they are a matter of common knowledge. All hail to these courageous pioneers, who fought for them during the years when they were most violently opposed!

The backgrounds of these two men were as different as can be imagined. Macfadden was an athlete who adopted vegetarianism and nature-cure methods because of their general value in building health. Dr. Tilden, on the other hand, had been for many years a regular physician (M.D.), giving drugs to his patients and treating them along orthodox medical lines until he became convinced that such methods were entirely fallacious. He then threw himself heart and soul into the promulgation of the nature-cure movement, contributing to it his experience, his wisdom and his wit, with the result that his influence began to be felt throughout the length and breadth of the land.

In the main, Tilden's teachings coincided with those of the earlier health reformers, particularly with those of Trall — who was, of course, also an M.D. But in some respects he extended them, and his special contribution consisted in emphasizing the all-importance of "toxemia," which he regarded as the basic and most fundamental causal factor in all so-called "diseases." If the patient suffers from toxemia, he is sick; rid him of his toxemia, and he is well. That was the key-note of his teachings, around which all else revolved. Years of experience only confirmed him in this belief.

"One of the first things to do to get rid of any so-called "disease," wrote Dr. Tilden, "is to get rid of toxemia; for it is this state of the blood that makes disease possible. Infection, drug and food-poisoning may kill; but if they do not, they will be short-lived in a subject free from enervation and toxemia. Conversely, the poison will linger in the system until Toxemia is overcome; then elimination will remove all traces of infection."

What, then, according to Tilden, is an acute disease? It is a "toxemic crisis;" a point where the body can no longer dispose of the excess. Something is then bound to happen. The liver begins to break down, the kidneys become blocked, the skin breaks out in an eruption, morbid matter is discharged from the mucous surfaces — as, e.g., when we have a "cold in the head." No matter what the outward symptoms may be, the inner cause is always the same — toxemia — which manifests its presence either in this way or in that. Remove this toxemia, and the patient recovers, no matter what his "disease" may be. The cause is the same; it is only the symptoms which vary.

How different is this conception from that maintained by the ordinary doctor! For him there are dozens — scores — of different "diseases," all malign, all largely mysterious, all having different causes, all requiring different treatment. He believes this because he has been so taught, and because he has mistaken the symptoms for the disease itself. Tell the average medical man that jaundice and Bright's Disease, and ear-ache, and arthritis, and mumps, and chicken-pox, and ulcers, and constipation, and a cold in the head, are all due to the same cause, and that all of them can easily be cured by the same methods, and he will probably froth at the mouth with rage, or regard you with cold contempt, as an utter ignoramus. And yet this is undoubtedly true, and can easily be proved true by treating the patient along simple, nature-cure lines, when he will recover in every case with similar ease and promptness. Toxemia is the basic cause of all these conditions, and when that cause is removed the patient recovers with relatively equal facility.

An "acute disease" is therefore merely a violent effort on the part of nature to expel toxic material; a "chronic disease" is a condition in which this underlying toxemia is constantly present. There is no fundamental difference between the two, save that the former represents a violent remedial effort, while the latter is a state of tolerance. As Dr. Page expressed it: "The various acute diseases, so-called, are in point of fact acute *remedies* for chronic *disease*." Due to the depletion of the vital energies, the system is unable, for the time being, to make the required effort. It therefore retains its toxins — and the patient is constantly ill.

In current medical literature, the terms "toxin" and "toxemia" are associated with "germs," and the excretions of germs — which are supposed to be responsible for the "disease" noted. This is not the sense in which the hygienist regards these terms. Not believing in the germ-theory of disease, he has a different concept. For him, toxemia consists in poisonous material which has found its way into the blood-stream and the body generally, from the bowel, as the result of over-eating and dietetic indiscretions. It is the "morbid matter" of the old health-reformers — with a new name

Again, it must be clearly understood that there are no such things as "local diseases." What are so classified are but the local manifestations of a general condition. Rectify that condition, and the local manifestation will disappear.

Once more, symptoms and "diseases" are considered by many to be virtually identical — as shown by their treatments. If the patient complains of pain over the region of the liver, then the liver is treated; if over the kidneys, then these organs are subjected to "suitable medication"; and so on. Purely local treatment is given. If the pain is relieved, and the symptoms temporarily disappear, the patient is thought to be "cured." Of course this is a complete fallacy. The liver is in trouble because some *cause* is at work, insuring its mal-functioning and giving rise to the symptoms noted. Remove this cause, and the symptoms disappear. Merely subduing pain, or relieving symptoms without removing this cause, will do the patient more harm than good. It gives him a false sense of security, while as a matter-of-fact he remains as sick a man as he was before. Practically the whole of the orthodox medical treatment is based upon this fundamental error — confusing symptoms with the causal factors underlying these symptoms. The only logical treatment consists in removing the cause, then the symptoms will cease. Inasmuch as toxemia is this fundamental cause, in practically all cases, it is obvious that its removal will bring about a return to normal health —no matter what the symptoms may be, or where located.

Dr. Tilden was strongly of the opinion that toxemia results mainly from over-eating, and eating the wrong kinds of food. He also believed that "enervation" is an important factor — since, if the nervous energies are low, the digestive and eliminative organs cannot properly perform their functions, and toxins begin to accumulate within the system. In this connection he says—

"Using energy in excess of normal production brings on enervation. Few people waste nerve-energy in one way only. Food is a stimulant. Overeating is over-stimulating. Add to this excess one or two other stimulants — coffee or tobacco — excessive venery, overwork and worry — and one subject to that amount of drain of nerve-energy will become decidedly enervated. Elimination falls far short of requirements; consequently toxin accumulates in the blood. This adds a pronounced auto-toxin stimulation to that coming from over-stimulating habits, and completes a vicious circle. This complex stands for a disease-producing Toxemia, which will be permanent except as toxin-crises (so-called acute diseases) lower the amount of toxin, again to accumulate and continue until the habits that keep the body enervated are controlled. Perfect health cannot be established until all enervating habits have been eliminated."

Enervation is thus due partly to physical and partly to mental causes. Toxemia is the main physical cause — though supplemented by other bad habits. The mental factors we shall come to later on in this booklet.

Tilden taught that without nerve-energy the functions of the various organs of the body cannot properly be carried on. Secretions are necessary for preparing the building-up material to take the place of worn-out tissue. The worn-out tissue must be removed — eliminated — from the blood as fast as it is formed, or it accumulates, and, as it is toxic, the system will be poisoned. This in turn becomes a source of enervation. Elimination of the waste-products of tissue-building is just as necessary as the building-up process. As these two important functions depend on each other, and as both depend on the proper amount of nerve-energy to do their work well, it behooves all people who would enjoy life and health to the full to understand in what way they may be frugal in using nerve-energy, so that they may learn to live conservatively and prudently, thereby enjoying the greatest mental and physical efficiency, and also the longest life.

When a man is seemingly well one day and sick (or dead) the next, what has happened? According to the orthodox medical point-of-view, he has "caught" a "disease," from which he is now suffering. According to the hygienist's point-of-view, however, something quite different has happened. Long-continued toxemia has finally resulted in a crisis being reached; the body is making a sudden and violent effort to expel the overload of poisons, and this has resulted in a set of symptoms, which are mistaken for a "disease." It is the last straw which has broken the camel's back! If a man is apparently well on Monday and has a cold in the head on Tuesday, one might be tempted to think that he had become ill over-night. As a matter of fact, the situation is precisely the reverse: the man's really dangerous state was on Monday; on Tuesday he has begun to get well! — since the body is now throwing-off the excess of toxic matter which it had formerly retained. The restorative effort is on; the man is on the road to recovery. But — holding the views he does — the average man at once begins to try and stifle the cold, to smother the symptoms, to stop the curative process at work! Instead of which he should aim at removing the *cause* of the cold — which is toxemia. This can most easily be accomplished by fasting, coupled with bathing, deep breathing and plenty of rest in bed. These simple measures will remove the cause in short order; and as the cause is removed the symptoms will disappear automatically. As the result of the cold the man is actually in far better health than he was before it. The cold was merely a curing process. Yet the market is flooded with "cures" for colds — and the doctors are still mystified as to its nature and causation!

Says Dr. Tilden ("Criticisms of the Practice of Medicine," p. 25):

"It is hard for the average person, or even physician, to accept the fact, which should be generally known, that there are very few well people; and it is harder yet for them to believe that the neighbor and friend, so round and plump, with a rich color and a keen relish for food and every enjoyment of life, is saturated with poison, and his bodily resistance is reduced so low that pneumonia is about to set in; or that his kidneys have been worked overtime to such an extent that they are about to take on disease; or that his capillaries have become so obstructed, causing such a hyperaemia of the internal organs, that their functioning is greatly impaired; or that the arterial pressure on the blood vessels of the brain is so great that they are on the verge of rupture; or that the heart is going down under the strain. . . . This description could be extended to take in every part of the body, and, without exaggeration, I might continue relating what is going on in the bodies of those who are commonly rated as the most robust in every community. The irony of the situation is that these people believe themselves to be in excellent health, and, if at any time they feel in doubt, all they have to do to reassure themselves and prove beyond the possibility of a doubt that they are in ideal health, is to apply to one of the old-line insurance companies for a policy, which is usually granted them without a question! Chronic toxemia is not even recognized by doctors, and is not known. It is a passive state, gradually brought on by the common abuses, such as overtaxing in work and play, over-eating, or eating improper foods, incompatible combinations, and either too much starch or too much meat, and often too much of both; all represent a gradual backing-up in the system of waste products. . . .''

Dr. Tilden taught that, when a normal person is infected, the infection will not be eliminated entirely until enervation and toxemia are overcome. Unless such patients are put to bed and fasted until elimination is completed, then fed properly, and taught how to eat within their limitations, and unless they are willing to give up all enervating habits, there is no hope of their ever getting really well.

"It is a crime to feed anything to the sick. No food should be given until all symptoms are gone; then fruit and vegetable juices (never any animal food)." Dr. Tilden was in favor of full enemas, so as to rid the lower bowel of all decomposing food; and in this he had the support of many nature-cure physicians. Theoretically, it seems most logical. . . . This is, however, a disputed point, and there are many hygienists today who contend that such measures are useless, or worse than useless — that "enemas are enemies," and that the benefits to be derived from them are fictitious. Dr. Shelton is of this opinion, as so is Dr. GianCursio and others who have had great experience especially in fasting cases. This is a point which the author of this little book does not feel called upon to settle. Much has been said on both sides; and the only counsel I feel justified in offering at this time is to recommend a study of these viewpoints pro and con. Certainly Dr. Tilden in his day was in favor of enemas and gastric lavages.

He was also in favor of air-baths, frequent bathing, and any measures which would increase the activity of the skin — contending that the skin is an important organ of elimination, and generally much neglected. In this, of course, he was in agreement with Dr. Trall and the majority of the older health reformers.

All of them, however, are agreed on the necessity of keeping the patient warm and quiet — preferably in bed.

"Without nerve-energy the functions of the body cannot be carried on properly," says Dr. Tilden. "Work and worry will soon end in flagging energy—enervation. Rest from habits that enervate is the only way to put nature in line for curing. Sleep and rest of body and mind are necessary to keep a sufficient supply of energy. Few people in active life rest enough."

Dr. Tilden was careful to point out, however, that enervation per se is not a disease. But, by causing a flagging of the elimination of tissue-waste, which is toxic, the blood becomes charged with toxin, and is called toxemia. "This is disease; and when the toxin accumulates beyond the toleration point, a crisis takes place; which means that the poison is being eliminated. This is called disease, but it is not. The only disease is toxemia, and what we call diseases are the symptoms produced by a forced elimination of toxins, largely through the mucous membranes."

Often, as time runs on, however, the system becomes more tolerant of toxins — though they are still there. We thus form what Dr. Tilden called "the catching-cold habit," which means that we manifest the signs of a cold on the slightest provocation; a slight draught of cold air will start it going — when this would be unnoticed by the ordinary person in good health. So-called chronic diseases are due to this constant retention, within the body, of toxic material, and if this is too long continued, organic changes begin to take place.

Poise and equanimity are important factors in the prevention of enervation. If this can be maintained — relaxation and freedom from worry — the body will cease to be tense; and nothing is more enervating than tenseness of the muscles. There is a constant wasting of energy, which results in enervation. This is manifested in many ways — by nervousness, irritability, sleeplessness, inability to concentrate, etc. It may also give rise to local symptoms, which are attributed to other causes, and treated as local "diseases." An example will make this clear.

A sensitive, insignificant pile-tumor will often set up such a tense state of the entire muscular system as to render the subject a confirmed invalid. Yet piles, especially in the initial stages, can easily be relieved. They are largely due to extreme contraction of the sphincter muscles, with tenseness of the entire body, and muscular fatigue. If the finger be introduced into the rectum very gently, so as not to cause pain to the patient, and pressure be exerted. at the same time giving the patient suggestions of relaxation, he will, in the course of half-an-hour or so, experience immense relief, manifested by relaxation of the sphincters and reduction of the piles. Tension is largely responsible for this condition.

Dr. Tilden contended that "fear is the greatest of all causes of enervation." Fears begin in childhood, and unwise parents are largely responsible for them. Orthodox religion, with its doctrines of hell-fire and brimstone, is also an important factor in the building of early fears. Confidence in Nature and her laws will do much to counteract these harmful teachings. Adults, too, are full of fears. Worries, business troubles, frustrations, and anxiety as to the future, are great devitalizers; financial insecurity is a tremendously important factor. Many fear old age, premature death and the "catching" of some "disease." A thorough understanding of the laws of nature and the true causation of so-called "diseases" would go far towards dispelling these fears.

Self-indulgence is another important factor in causing enervation, and so are over-work and boredom. Grief, shock, anger, egotism, selfishness, envy and jealousy: these and similar emotions all serve to induce enervation — and hence toxemia.

In stressing the importance and influence of these devastating emotions, Dr. Tilden had a great advantage over the old-time health reformers, for in their day psychiatry was almost unknown, psychology still in its infancy, and little was known concerning the effects of fear and similar emotional states. He was therefore able to take advantage of these newer findings, as well as "suggestion" and the improved psychotherapeutic technic. At the same time, his writings (in the opinion of the present writer, at least) fall far short of those of Trall, Graham and others in scope and philosophical insight. There is an enormous amount of repetition in his books and his various writings; he emphasizes the same points over and over again, using other words, and they are at times discursive and meandering, not keeping to the main point, but coming back to it after some extensive and more or less unrelated side-issue. This is not to be found in the writings of the "old masters." Trall especially was concise and to the point. A further criticism might be that Dr. Tilden was rather inclined to monopolize full credit for his expositions, paying scant attention to the previous work of others. These are perhaps understandable human frailties; at the same time they somewhat detract from the historic value of his writings. In spite of this, of course, it must be admitted that Dr. Tilden did an enormous amount of good, in spreading these doctrines, and in influencing the trend of thinking in the public mind. His influence was extensive, and important. Certainly his books should be in the library of every true health-reformer or exponent of the older nature-cure.

Naturally, Dr. Tilden was opposed to the craze for operations, and also to vaccination, serum-therapy and the germ-theory of disease. These are all based upon the fundamental medical fallacy — that disease, so-called, is a harmful entity which has somehow entered the body of the patient, and must be expelled. These systems confuse cause and effect, symptoms with the cause of those symptoms, a restorative and remedial effort for a malign entity. All of them fail to realize the true nature of our various "diseases." They fail to grasp the fundamental unity and oneness of disease, or perceive what really happens when the patient is "cured." All of them fail to see that certain concomitant factors — such as germs — are not necessarily *causal* factors, but are merely coincidental. Lacking this knowledge, and a true realization of the "action" of drugs — so clearly enunciated in the writings of Trall — it is only natural that the medical profession, *en masse,* should have placed the cart before the horse, and done everything (to use the slang of the day)—backwards. Only a complete right-about-face can rectify this situation and convert the "science of medicine" into a "true healing art."

In an article in the "Health Review and Critique," (Dec., 1936), Dr. Tilden said:

"In acute diseases we see nature making her most profound efforts at getting rid of poison. . . . Toxemic subjects, on account of having less resistance, are susceptible to food-poisoning. Indeed, these subjects have a limited digestive capacity, and they are often poisoned by decomposition of the food they eat. This is autoinfection—self-poisoning. Typhoid fever, pneumonia, appendicitis, and other diseases of an auto-infectious character, are clearly cases of auto-infection. The toxemic subject has so little resistance that when his digestion is crowded beyond its capacity, decomposition takes place, and, if not discovered and corrected, it will cause a disease to develop of the character of those named. . . .

"The treatment I advocate cannot be accepted so long as the profession clings to the delusive idea the disease *can be cured* . . . . That disease primarily originates in bad habits cannot be gainsaid. If health stands for anything, it is an ideal physiological state of body and mind. Health means a normal physiology—a normal body, the organs of which are all working in harmony with each other, the secretions and excretions of which are balanced; a physiology in which the mind and body are poised. In other words, health represents a body and mind adjusted to, and in unison with, the physical and psychical laws of nature. And disease represents any departure from this ideal state. . . .

"It may be asked, 'Does your system cure everybody? Will no one die if all adopt your plan?' My plan will not create new organs, nor prevent the body from dying when one or more of its important organs are completely out-of-commission from disorganization. Degeneration of vital organs carried beyond the point where coming-back-to the normal is possible, means that life will end from forced organic dissolution. Life depends upon organic harmony. As long as disease is functional, every case will recover when the cause of the functional derangement is removed. Where organic change is not too great, removing the cause, and keeping it removed, will allow the organ to return to the normal."

(By "my plan" Dr. Tilden really means the plan advocated by hygienists everywhere. His language in the above passage is also loose, in speaking of "disease" as he does. However, he is using popular language and his meaning is of course clear).

Many of Dr. Tilden's books and writings are devoted to specific ailments, which he lists more or less alphabetically. He often shows the inter-relationship of these conditions, and how seemingly different and distinct afflictions are basically one and the same, only different organs and symptoms being involved. The same cause is always there, and the same methods will suffice in every one of them. The very simplicity of the hygienic system proves the greatest obstacle to its acceptance! People, and particularly medical men, simply "cannot believe it." Moreover, it must be remembered that the majority of people are so thoughtless, so lazy and so self-indulgent, that they will not consent to reform their lives in any respect, preferring to buy health in a bottle! It is so much easier! The only trouble is that such a method never works, and that the same trouble recurs a little later, or some other trouble which is even worse — though of course the two are never associated in such a person's mind. Yet it is the same cause, taking now one channel and now another, which is always at work. Only the removal of this cause can bring true relief.

A sample illustration will perhaps serve to show this inter-relationship, and the simplicity of the theory and methods employed. Speaking of one of the commonest of all disorders, Dr. Tilden says:

"The real cause of arthritis is Toxemia, brought about by faulty diet and enervating habits of living, and it is the correction of these that makes the relief or cure of the condition possible in almost every case. With toxemia removed, *no case* is too far gone for improvement to be made and maintained. . . . The results obtained by the therapeutic fast (fast with water only) or corrective eliminative diet (usually fruit juices) are often spectacular. Pain usually diminishes rapidly and mobility of affected joints increases as toxemia is overcome. The progressively destructive effects of the condition are arrested, and joints, muscles and nerves lose their irritation and tension, and the way is paved for the restorative measures of correct diet, massage and exercise. Lumbago, neuritis, sciatica, neuralgia, and muscular rheumatism are soon overcome with the definite assurance that they *will not recur* at a later date or develop into arthritis."

Dr. Tilden led an intensely active life, and spread his ideas through various channels. Beginning with his little magazine "The Stuffed Club," this later developed into the "Philosophy of Health," and this again into the "Health Review and Critique." He supervised his Health Institute in Denver, and carried on an enormous practice, both individually and by mail. He also wrote a number of books, the best known of these being:

Diseases of Women and Easy Childbirth.
Toxemia Explained.
Tilden Cook Book.
Children: Their Health and Happiness.
Constipation.
Cholera Infantum.
Criticisms of the Practice of Medicine (2 vols.)
Impaired Health (2 vols.)
Epigrams (2 vols.)
Appendicitis.
The Pocket Dietition: Food (2 vols.)
Typhoid Fever.
Venereal Diseases.

As might be expected, Dr. Tilden was of the opinion that babies are usually fed too often and too much — thus laying the foundations for a later chronic toxemia. In this he agrees with Dr. Charles E. Page, who contended (in his "How to Feed the Baby"), that three daily feedings were sufficient, and stated that he brought-up his own baby on this regime, and that it remained entirely free from the complaints common to infants. Dr. Tilden was not as radical as this, believing that the baby should be fed every four hours, but that it should not be awakened for the purpose of feeding, if it was asleep. It should be kept quiet and free from undue excitement.

Children are, as a rule, notoriously over-fed, and it is for this very reason that "children's diseases" are so common. There is no reason why a child should ever become ill (no matter how much it is "exposed to contagion"), and if it is not toxemic it will never suffer from any of the illnesses of childhood. Many hygienists have reared their children along rational lines, without one of them ever having a serious illness. This record should be universal, if their nutrition were properly managed, and they were taught how to live normal, healthful lives.

As a matter-of-fact, this perverted nutrition begins even before birth —in the food-habits of the pregnant mother. There is no greater delusion on earth than the old adage that she must "eat for two." The fallacy of this idea may easily be shown. Suppose the baby weighs nine pounds at birth. This represents approximately a pound a month, or half-an-ounce a day This is all the extra food necessary. But women are urged to eat one and two and three extra pounds of food a day—to supply the expected infant with plenty of nourishment! Is it any wonder that women have such a time at childbirth, and that lacerations and other complications occur—their tissues being shot through-and-through with toxemia and fatty-tissue? Besides, such over-sized babies are abnormal. Dr. Tilden contended that the normal child, at birth, should not weigh more than three or four pounds — which would render birth relatively easy, and prevent the complications so often noted. The average woman prides herself on the weight of her baby—the more the better! This is a complete delusion, only rendered possible by the false ideas so universally prevalent. Normal growth should be slow but sure.

This groundwork having been laid, example and habit carry it still further. The child is often urged to eat, under the mistaken idea that he must do so, in order to "keep up his strength." Nature tells him not to eat, and he may even have an aversion for food; but he is urged to eat nevertheless. All hygienists know that this is one of the greatest crimes that can be committed (physiologically); for nature (like mother) knows best!

The same false ideas are to be noted in the treatment of invalids. Special "Menus" are prepared, so as to "tempt the appetite," whereas what is needed more than anything else is a fast. This practice is doubtless responsible for most of the "relapses" and "complications" which are so often noted, rather than a steady progress towards health. The sicker the patient, the more essential it is that he should fast, being allowed at best only a few simple fruit-juices. But nothing equals a water-fast; and Dr. Tilden was among the first to advocate this—though few of his patients were ever placed on a prolonged fast, so far as I can discover. (In this, however, I may be in error.)

It must always be remembered that food eaten at such times does not nourish the patient; on the contrary it merely weakens and poisons him, thereby adding to his toxemia. If too much coal is already on the fire, the way to make it burn more brightly is not to heap more coal upon it, but to clean-out the clinkers and turn-on a forced draught. Similarly, the human body needs time for elimination and rest, and this can best be supplied by placing the patient on a fast, thereby allowing it time, and giving it the opportunity, to dispose of the over-load of impurities it already possesses.

The sick patient continues to waste-away, as a rule, no matter whether he eats or not; as a matter of fact, he becomes thinner and weaker if food be administered. There is no greater delusion in the world than the idea that food "gives strength," at such times, for it has precisely the opposite effect. The patient will recover his health and strength far more rapidly without food than with it. This has been demonstrated thousands of times, and is being proved every day by hygienists everywhere. Overeating is to blame for 99 percent of our illnesses.

Says Dr. Tilden:

"The most powerful eliminant is a fast. In other words, give nature a rest, and she needs no so-called 'cures.' Rest means: stay in bed, poised mind and body, and fast. Nature then works without handicaps, unless fear is created by the old fear-mongers, professional and lay, sending to the patient the warning, 'It is dangerous to fast; you will never live through it.' These wiseacres do not know that there is a vast difference between fasting and starving."

All so-called "disease," then, according to the Tilden philosophy, is the result of toxemia, and this in turn is due largely to enervation, which prevents active and proper elimination. Restore the patient's energy-level, rid him of his toxemia, and he will invariably get well. The philosophy of health is simple, when rightly understood. Yet it is in conformity with common-sense and the laws of Nature. Conform to these laws, and lasting health will be yours! These are basic elements of Dr. Tilden's teachings. In his life, they were proved by the treatment of thousands of others. Some day, Dr. Tilden will doubtless be regarded as one of the great benefactors of humanity, worthy of a place in the Hall of Fame, together with other great health-reformers. And there are indications that this day is not far distant!

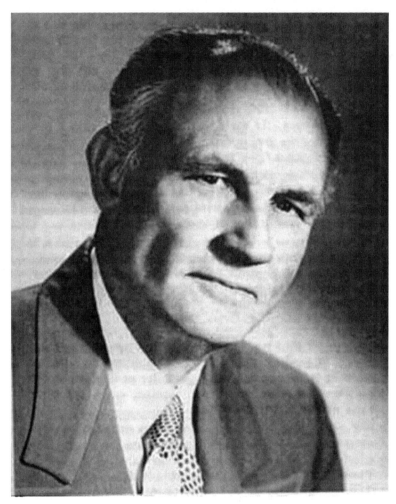

Yours for Health Truth
Herbert M. Shelton

Principles of Natural Hygiene

By Herbert M. Shelton, N. D., as printed in *Dr. Shelton's*
Hygienic Review, 1949.

The Hygienic System not only introduced a *materia hygienica* and a new practice, but also a new theory and philosophy in biological science that is at variance with and in opposition to all the fundamental doctrines and dogmas on which all medical systems, past and present, have been founded. It claims to have ignored the false principles of the old schools (and of the new) and to have based its philosophy and its practice upon the unerring and demonstrable laws of nature. The principles and practices of the hygienic school are comparatively new, original and independent. They have never been written in medical books, nor taught in medical schools, nor recognized by the medical profession. While they are each and all in direct opposition to each and all of the fundamental principles on which the popular medical systems are based, they are demonstrably in harmony with the laws of nature.

The *Hygienic System* not only rejects wholly and totally, as both unnecessary and injurious, each and all of the poisons known to the *materia medicas* of the medical schools as drug-remedies, but it also rejects the philosophy or theories on which their employment is predicated. *Hygiene* controverts all their fundamental dogmas, denies all their pretended science, challenges all of their philosophy, and condemns nearly all of their practices.

Let me begin by defining my subject. *Hygiene* is that branch of biology which investigates and applies the conditions upon which life and health depend, and the means by which health is sustained in all its virtue and purity, and restored when it has been lost. *Hygiene* is not a system of therapeutics. It professes to build health in all forms of diseased states by the employment of hygienic agents alone and without the employment of poisons or resort to enervating palliatives of any nature. Constructive surgery forms the only non-hygienic measure ever endorsed by the natural hygienist.

A true hygiene is not empirical, but rests upon the immutable and unchanging laws of nature. All real science comes from recognition of the laws of nature. These are the principles which embody all truth, and whose proper arrangement into a system constitutes all science, and art is but the application of these truths to uses, to the production of the desired results.

The laws of nature, the truths of the universe, the principles of science, are just as certain, as fixed and immutable in their relations to human organization, in relation to life, in relation to health, in relation to happiness, in relation to disease, as they are in relation to all things else.

Because man has not studied himself aright he knows not the laws of his own being. Instead of looking to the laws of nature for enlightenment he has gone in pursuit of strange gods, and become the worshipper of idols, and the victim of his own folly. He has sought to understand the ways of evil instead of good, he has studied the "laws of disease" rather than the philosophy of health, he has seated disorder on the throne of the universe, and in trying to adapt himself to this king, he has been led into a thousand foolish fashions, perpetrated innumerable violations of the laws of order, and brought upon himself inconceivable miseries so that we may say of mankind personified:

"Sickness sits caverned in his hollow eye."

Health is nothing more than life in a normal state because of normal conditions; while disease is life in an abnormal state because of abnormal conditions   Here is a very simple, but entirely correct definition of disease; it is abnormal vital action.

What is necessary to the production of a living thing is also necessary to its preservation. The human body is developed under certain natural conditions and influences, and by the use of certain natural agents and materials, and these same conditions and influences and materials are essential and all that are essential to its maintenance in a state of health. What causes a human being to grow into manhood or womanhood in health and vigor is necessary to preserve that health and vigor, and all that is necessary.

A rational hygienist will study and understand exactly and precisely the nature and influences of air, water, food, light, exercise, rest, sleep, temperature, clothing, housing, noise, the emotions, etc., and apply the knowledge daily, hourly, constantly, acting ever and always in proper relation to the laws of life, to the preservation and restoration of health. What is needed is a complete system of hygiene, not an exaggerated attention given to but one hygienic factor. Not exercise alone, not diet alone, not sunshine alone, not emotional poise alone, not any one factor alone: but a well-rounded, correlated and integrated system, which includes all the conditions and materials of healthy life. Health must be built and maintained as a unit and must rest upon the total mode of living.

In its widest sense, hygiene is the application of the principles of nature to the preservation and restoration of health. Applied to the sick, it consists in finding the cause of the patient's suffering and removing this, and in restoring to the patient the conditions of a healthy life. This is accomplished by teaching him how to prepare and eat a proper diet, secure abundance of fresh air, to use sunshine properly, how to exercise, rest, clothe himself properly etc. It may be said to be a system of purification, vivification and rejuvenation. By the use of agents and conditions that are normal to the body the system is cleansed, invigorated and restored to healthy action

Health and disease are not accidents, but developments of law. Just as the same law of gravity ca ries a balloon upward under one set of conditions and brings it back to earth under another, or floats a ship under one set of conditions and sinks it under another, just as it is the same chemical affinity that preserves a stick of dynamite under one set of conditions and explodes it under another, so the same law of life produces health under one set of conditions and disease under another. A knowledge of the laws of life makes health and disease matters of our own choice. We can have the one or the other as we supply the conditions for the one or the other.

The *Hygienic System* was the first and, so far, the only school that makes the laws of nature and the conditions of health its chief reliance in the preservation and restoration of health. These are taught in no other school on earth save the *Hygienic*. Nor are they proclaimed to be taught in any other. On these points, we speak advisedly.

For three thousand years medical men, philosophers and scientists of the highest abilities have sought an understanding of the essential nature of disease, the mode of action of drugs, the precise relation of drugs to disease and the healing power of nature. Today disease is listed as one of the "seven modern mysteries." Most of the standard works on pharmacology contain brief efforts at explaining the *modus operandi* of drug action, but none of these are satisfactory. How drugs act is still as much a mystery as the nature of disease itself. No one pretends to understand the relation of drugs to disease; there seems to be little understanding of the healing power of nature and disease and the healing powers are still, as they were in the days of Hippocrates, thought of as antagonistic forces or processes.

Confessing that they do not know the essential nature of any disease, medical men are incessantly drugging all disease, as though they know all about it. Confessing their lack of knowledge of the *modus operandi* of any drug they are incessantly using thousands of them as though the actions of all of them are known.

How can a successful means of dealing with anything be devised when the thing is not understood? If they do not know the essence of disease and do not understand its nature, how can they build a successful method of treating the sick? A knowledge of the essential nature of disease must be at the very foundation of any truly scientific care of the sick. To attempt to operate a locomotive, while one is unacquainted with the power of steam, would be rash; but to treat sick people, while ignorant of the nature and cause of disease, as medical men acknowledge they are, is madness, even to insanity. He who cannot make one blade of grass to grow may destroy millions.

Now *Hygienists* do profess to understand the nature of disease and the apparent actions of drugs, and understanding these things they reject all drugs.

Disease is as much a vital process as is health. Health is vital action in the construction and conservation of bodily organs, and disease is vital action in defense and reparation of the same organs. Health is the normal play of all the vital functions, disease is remedial effort, or their abnormal play. The difference between health and disease is simply this: Health is the regular and normal performance of the functions of the body; it is normal action — physiology; disease is irregular and abnormal action — pathology. Health expresses the aggregate of vital actions and processes that nourish and develop the body and all its organs and structures and provide for reproduction; in other words, health is the action of the vital powers in building up and replenishing the organic structures; or in still plainer words, the conversion of the elements of food into the elements of the body's tissues, and the elimination of waste. Disease is the aggregate of vital actions and processes by which poisons are expelled and damages repaired; it is the action of the same powers that are active in health, in defending the organism against injurious or abnormal agencies and conditions.

To illustrate these two principles: the body does not act upon alcohol as it does upon food. It digests, absorbs, circulates, assimilates and uses food. It does not digest and assimilate alcohol. Alcohol is absorbed and circulated, but it is not appropriated. It is not used. The body acts against it, to resist it, to expel it, as it does all other poisons The normal work of digesting food is healthy action; the abnormal work of resisting and expelling alcohol is diseased action.

And thus the healing power of nature, the nature of which has been sought since the days of Hippocrates, and disease turn out to be one and the same thing. A partial recognition of this fact is implied in the belated admission by pathologists, of the constructive character of inflammation and the beneficial character of fever.

The healing principle is always in the living system itself. All living organisms are self-constructing, self-defending and self-repairing. The only power that can heal is the power that repairs; the only power that can repair is the power that produces; the power that now produces, repairs, heals, etc., is the power that is originally produced. The power that evolved a full-grown man from a fertilized ovum is the only healing power. It is an intrinsic, not an extrinsic power. The power that produced the organism is in it to maintain it.

The power which brought us into being, which causes us to grow through the various stages of development to manhood or womanhood also repairs the organism, sustains its growth, performs its functions heals its lesions — in a word, this power constitutes the only healing, repairing, preserving force. Huxley's "Hidden Artist," that made and fashioned the organs and the organism, is always on hand to continue its work in growth and repair and in function. In every living organism the process of repair is the process of reproduction, the same power which brought it into existence; is the same power that performs all the functions of life. It is folly to think some outside power can perform the functions of life.

It is by cell reproduction that repair takes place and this is not the work of any extrinsic agent or force, but of the inherent, intrinsic power of life. Nobody doubts that it is the same power that brought us into being that heals in the case of a wound. A surgeon would not think of opening the abdomen of a patient, if he was not certain that the processes of life would heal the wound thus inflicted. For he knows that he possesses no curative agencies that can heal a wound. Just why we insist upon thinking that some other agency than that of the powers of life are requisite in the healing of disease, in those cases where the causes of the trouble are not obvious, is hard to explain.

Healing is a process of evolution just as birth, growth and development are. Neither medicines, water, food, exercise, nor anything else external to the organism have any healing power. The same power that brought a man into health keeps him in health, and it alone can restore him to health. That power resides in the man, and nowhere else in nature. The same powers and processes of life are in operation in disease as in health. In disease, no new or extra-vital power is superadded to the processes of life.

Let me now explain the apparent actions of drugs. Observations of the phenomena that follow the use of a drug demonstrate that certain effects follow. But why they follow, how they follow, and what is their real cause, as distinct from their occasion, have not been determined. Until we know what cause produces a given effect we cannot explain the effect. As nobody has ever explained how drugs act on the body we offer this opposite explanation—that the living system acts on the drug. On the basis of this theory we find the explanation of most of the so-called effects of drugs and, we believe, that in time, all the other so-called actions will be explained on this basis. Whatever principle will explain the *modus operandi* of one poison will explain the *modus operandi* of them all.

We find the explanation of what are mistakenly called the actions of drugs in the laws of organization — in physiology rather than in chemistry or physics. Life and its variable phenomena furnish the proper field of inquiry. On the basis of such investigations we deny that drugs act at all, but insist that as lifeless, inorganic substances, they are as passive, inert, quiescent, and inactive when taken into the body as when resting in their various bottles on the druggist's shelves. They are acted upon, but do not act.

The *Hygienic* philosophy reduces this mysterious problem to a single truism, by reference to the primary premise — the law of relation between organic and inorganic matter. The law that applies to this problem is that in the relations between living and lifeless matter, living matter is active, lifeless matter is passive always. Medicines do not act at all. Lifeless matter, we reiterate, does not act on the living. This is the universal law in the relations of the living organism to everything that surrounds it. The drug in the stomach, the poison in the blood, the 'medicine' in the drug store, the food on the table, the water in the pitcher — these are all passive in their relations to the living organism. The organism acts upon all these things, either to appropriate them or to reject them and expel them. Drugs are lifeless, inorganic, inert substances and have no relation to the living save that of inertia, the same as a dry stick or a stone and since the incapacity to act is an inseparable characteristic of all lifeless matter, while, on the other hand, action is an inseparable characteristic of life, we know that whenever action takes place between living and lifeless matter, the former and not the latter, does the acting; they do nothing. They are done unto. They are acted upon. The living thing is active and the lifeless thing is passive. This is no denial of the mechanical actions of masses of matter, nor of the chemical actions of atoms of matter. We deny only that drugs have the actions — physiological, medicinal, etc. — attributed to them by pharmacologists and physicians.

Our main position, in general terms, may be thus stated: The symptoms or phenomena which result when a drug-remedy is taken into the system are the evidences of vital resistance to the drug (the action of the system against the drug contemplating its expulsion) and are not evidences of the remedial action of the drug on the body, as is commonly supposed. The law can be demonstrated and we think that it may be best expressed about as follows: *The resident forces in the various tissues, acting preservatively, give rise to all the phenomena that are mistaken for the actions of drugs.* It is *modus operandi* of the living organism. The *modus operandi* of drugs is a misnomer. On the basis of the various medical theories that have been offered to account for "drug action," it is impossible to give the rationale of the "action" of any drug. On the *Hygienic* theory it is possible to explain the rationale of all of them. The rationale of the effects of all "medicines" is inseparably connected with life. Whatever will explain the *modus operandi* of one "medicine" or one poison will explain the *modus operandi* of all of them. Two separate and distinct principles of action are not admissable.

This is either true or false. If true, the whole system of administering drugs to cure disease ought to be abandoned as unsound in science and injurious in results. All drug remedies are absolutely poisonous. This difference of principle involves the essential philosophy of drug-medication in all its schools, modes, phases, and modifications. The point on which we differ comes to the veritable explanation, the rationale, of all remedial or medicinal agents.

Medical men in all ages have mistaken the actions of the living organism in self-defense for the actions of foreign substances upon it. They have mistaken the vital action in expelling foreign substances from the body for an attack of some outside entity upon the body. In thus mistaking the true nature of operations seen in disease, they have attempted to subdue, suppress and destroy the very actions and processes that alone can save the life of the patient. In their efforts to cure (exorcise or kill an imaginary enemy) they have been warring upon the human constitution. All the importance attached to the management of the sick with drugs comes from a non-recognition of these principles, from a mistake in regard to the essential nature of the actions that follow the taking of poisons.

The philosophy of *Hygienic* care of the sick is predicated on the primary premise that those things which are constitutionally adapted to the preservation of health are also the proper things to use in restoring health. The same agents and conditions that have been found necessary to the enjoyment of health are also best calculated to enable the body to overcome and remove unhealthy conditions within.

All healing power is inherent in the living organism and all true remedial agents (materials, influences, processes) must harmonize with the laws of life and must be susceptible of constructive use by the organism. No substance can be used remedially which bears no normal relation to the organism. All the "remedial agents" have normal or physiological relations to the living organism. They may be used constructively to preserve health, or remedially to restore health, but they are not cures. They may be abused and that abuse causes disease.

In the class of *Hygienic* agencies can be included only the actual necessities of life — food, air, water, sunlight, rest, sleep, relaxation, exercise, play, warmth, cleanliness, hope, faith, courage — and the means of securing these. For three thousand years these were classed as non-naturals. They were either rejected entirely or ignored in practice. Drugs were classed as naturals.

None of the real *Hygienic* materials and conditions can be dispensed with permanently. Such is the inherent nature of the truly *Hygienic* factors that their employment affords an actual compensation for the energy expended in their appropriation by the organism; a truly *Hygienic* agent and influence gives and does not merely take. Rightly used it gives more than it takes. Only when abused does it take more than it gives.

All too many people think of *Hygienic* agencies and conditions as limited in their work to the preservation of health. They think that, while *Hygiene* is good for the person in health, it is weak and unreliable in a state of sickness. When sick we need more potent, more powerful "remedies" — poisons — that in health we do not need. In fact, it is well-known that if a healthy person takes poison it will make him sick. We have, here, a strange perversion of truth and a strange anomaly of logic. Things that are good for the healthy are not good for the sick; things that are bad for the healthy are good for the sick.

Hygienists reject poisons. Indeed, the *Hygienists* are the only ones who have persistently and consistently rejected all poisons. Are poisons, then, *Hygienic* agencies? To believe in the necessity of any substance, or condition, we must have evidence that these are beneficial if used habitually in a state of health, that their use will effect some necessary result in a state of health. They must be indispensable to life. If drugs are *Hygienic* agencies they are actual necessities of life and their uses are not to be confined to times of illness alone. They are essential in health as well as in disease. To believe that they are *Hygienic* factors, we must believe that they are essential to effecting some necessary result in a state of health, and to regard them as *Hygienic* agents we must believe that the habitual use of them by a person in health would be beneficial.

Everything is poisonous which the system rebels against and rejects in a state of health. Everything is *Hygienic* which it seeks, uses and appropriates. Drugs are non-usable substances; they do not nourish the tissues, they cannot be transformed into blood and tissue, they cannot invigorate the body or any part of it, they cannot be used in any manner in the performance of any of the normal functions of life, nor in the performance of any of the abnormal actions of life, hence they must be expelled. They can only occasion vital resistance, hence their use results in a waste of vital power. They are definitely un-*hygienic* and opposed to all the vital interests of life.

Science gives us no grounds for including poisonous agents among *Hygienic* agents. No one supposes that poisons (drugs) are necessary in a state of health, that they are necessities of life, or that their use produces any necessary or beneficial result in a state of health. Drugs (and many other agents) employed in the treatment of the sick have nothing in their nature that can afford any compensation to the organism for the energy employed in resisting and expelling them. It is only in a state of impaired health that their use is supposed to be needed. But if poisons cannot be beneficial in a state of health, they cannot be helpful in a state of sickness. If all truly remedial agents have normal or physiological relations to the living organism, as *Hygienists* proclaim, then drugs of every kind cannot be classed as "remedial agents."

Should the sick be poisoned? That is a startling question. If our people had not been so badly miseducated this question could be answered by asking: should the well be poisoned? For there is no more reason why a sick man should be poisoned than a well man. No physician has ever been able to give a rational theory, or even a plausible hypothesis, or even the shadow of a shade of an argument, why any person, because he is sick, should take into his body a poison that would certainly induce disease in a well person.

Everybody seems to know.that drug-medicines are poisons; that they are always injurious to persons in health. All persons are very careful to exclude them from their victuals and drink. They seem to be aware that if, by accident or design, they take them into the system while it is in health, sickness will be the consequence. What person would dare to take an ordinary dose of calomel, or antimony while in perfect health? Yet, let him get sick, and he swallows them, not only without fear, but as the essential conditions of safety. We suspect, indeed, we know, there is a terrible delusion abroad on this subject.

It is a strange practice that a remedy which always tends to kill is chosen to cure the sick. If poison be both our bane and our boon, we are indeed strangely made. In the days when physicians bled patients to cure them and butchers bled pigs to kill them, and gave arsenic to patients to cure them, while farmers fed arsenic to rats to kill them, a sick rat might refuse to eat arsenic because it kills well rats, but a sick man could not exercise so much intelligence.

It is not true that things which are poisonous in health become innocuous in disease. Nothing changes its relation to the human organism because this is sick or well. A food or a poison is so once and always— under all possible circumstances. Bread will never corrode the tissues and calomel will never nourish them, be the conditions of health or the circumstances of disease what they may.

The idea of poisoning a person because he is sick is founded on a false notion of the nature of disease. Disease is regarded, in all teachings of the medical books, as a something foreign to the organism, as an enemy; and poisons are given to war upon and destroy the enemy. But as the truth happens to be the exact contrary, all this poisoning business happens to be exactly wrong—nothing more nor less than a war on human constitutions.

There are better ways of caring for the sick than that of poisoning them. They need helpful, not hurtful things. It will amaze the uninitiated to watch the body and see what it can do for itself in the way of recovery if left uncrippled by drugs of any kind, in large or small doses.

History reveals to us that the theory that the earth revolves on its axis was controverted for twelve hundred years before it was finally accepted. It was so preposterous and absurd to the people who knew that the earth is flat and that the sun goes under and around the earth once in twenty-four hours, that they could not accept it. In like manner, it is difficult to get people to accept the simple truism that *Hygienic* agents, that is, agents adapted to health, are better for the sick than pathogenic agents, that is, agents that induce sickness in the well.

Getting along in sickness without drugs of some kind has a strange sound to most of us when we first hear of it. The idea of caring for the sick with poisons has become deeply ingrained in us. Most of us are "born with it." It has grown with our growth and strengthened with our strength. It has been associated with all our thoughts, observations and experiences on the subject of caring for the sick. This is the reason that we must be in some measure, at least, un-educated and re-educated. Getting along without drugs may seem as preposterous as did the theory that the earth rotates on its axis and revolves around the sun, to the ancient astronomers. Yet some of the most remarkable recoveries on record have occurred without medical treatment of any kind. The great error of physicians has been that of attributing recovery to the operations of their poisons, while they have left out of account the healing powers of the body itself.

Hygienists are not engaged in curing disease. Indeed, we hold that all efforts to cure disease are based upon false notions of the essential nature of disease.

Disease is a process of purification and reparation. It is not an enemy of the vital powers but a struggle of the vital powers themselves in self-defense. We of the *Hygienic* school do not regard the diseases which are said to kill so many every year as of themselves, dangerous; we hold that the great mortality seen in these diseases is due to suppressive and combative treatment. Disease is not a thing to be removed, expelled, subdued, broken up, destroyed, conquered, or cured or killed. It is not a thing, but an action; not an entity, but a process; not an enemy at war with the living organism, but a remedial effort; not a substance to be opposed, but an action to be cooperated with.

The *Hygienic System* is not a collection of therapies and cures. Nor are *Hygienists* engaged in a ceaseless search after new, more novel, ever more sensational, and miraculous cures. In the whole history of the *Hygienic* movement, not a single one of its practitioners has brought forth a single cure. No rapid succession of wonder-cures from *Hygienic* sources, each to enjoy its brief day in the sun, only to pass into that long night that is followed by no sunrise. *Hygienists* go all the way in this matter. We have no "curative agencies" and recognize none. Disease is the result of violation of physiological law and a return to obedience is the condition of recovery.

Why experiment with a host of "remedies?" Why not study cause and effect? Only by removing the causes that have impaired the functions of life can a normal function be restored. This requires, first of all, a full and thorough correction of the habits and conditions of life.

The principles of the *Hygienic System* are true, hence, if they are understood they will be believed; and if they are intelligently believed, they will be successfully practiced; for the whole of *Hygienic* art, both in health and sickness, is merely the application of scientific principles to the varying curcumstances of life, (of health and disease) and, in sickness, to the constantly changing conditions of the patient. *Hygienic* methods are not empirical, they are not experimental, they are not haphazardous and they are not to be employed haphazardly. The *Hygienic System* is established upon a settled and scientific basis, having fixed principles to guide the employment of all of its measures. Every particular process must conform to the principles of the system and all results are the results of unvarying accuracy.

The present much ado about psychosomatic medicine and about treating the whole man, the patient, instead of the disease is not new to *Hygienists*. We approach the matter from an entirely different angle than that of the physician and pseudo-psychologist, but caring for the whole man has been *Hygienic* practice from its beginning. Over a hundred years ago Sylvester Graham wrote: "If we could correctly understand the science of physiology or pathology, we must take into view, and thoroughly investigate, the whole nature and condition and relations of man—he who treats of the functions of the human organs, and the diseases of the human body, without fully and accurately considering the modifying influences of the mind, and of the various physical and moral circumstances acting on the healthy and on the morbid sensibilities and sympathies of the system, may indeed form a theory which will have its day of popular acceptance, but fortunate without a parallel will it be, if it does not, sooner or later, prove to possess sufficient error to sink it into utter disrepute, if not total oblivion."

The pioneer *Hygienists* held that the "physical, mental, moral and spiritual" parts of man are "parts of one stupendous whole, of one grand personality." They said very forcefully that the *Hygienist* must not look only to physical health, but that the "mental, moral and spiritual health of the individual, of the collective man," is his legitimate scope. Resorting to scriptural phraseology, which the earlier *Hygienists* frequently did, they pointed out that the physical, mental, moral and spiritual phases of man are all "members of one another," and that "if one member suffers all the members suffer with it, or if one member be honored, all the members rejoice with it."

For full health a complete and well-rounded program of physiological and biological living is essential. Health can only be produced as a unit and the total health program must meet all of the needs of life.

We are beginning to inquire, not how shall we get well, but, how shall we keep well. This is a wholesome change in public attitude towards health which has resulted directly from the work of the *Hygienists*. As important as *Hygienic* principles may be in giving the world better methods of caring for the sick, this is not the greatest benefit they are destined to confer upon the race. Far more important is their influence in preventing disease. An appreciation of *Hygienic* principles results in the understanding that in order to preserve health, the causes of disease must be avoided. This implies living in conformity with organic law and in all things, "cease to do evil and learn to do good."

Economy alone should cause people to adopt the *Hygienic System*. Its universal adoption by the people of the United States would save in physicians' bills, nursing bills, hospital bills, etc., alone, several hundred millions of dollars a year. An equal sum would be saved by avoiding loss of time from work or business. The enormous tax burden that the people bear to maintain public health organizations would be lifted from their shoulders. This enormous saving of money is small compared to the saving from suffering its adoption would assure.

Health is pre-eminently the great want of the age. A precise, intimate and practical knowledge of its conditions, and of the circumstances which induce disease, as well as of the way to remove diseases without incurring other evils as great, or worse, is the great need of the people. We believe the physical salvation of the human race depends on it.

As we understand the ways of nature and man, and the ways of man toward himself, all those examples of abnormal activity called disease and all premature deaths not caused by violence, are due to habits and practices perfectly explainable and as perfectly avoidable. And so believing, we cannot feel nor think that the physician, practitioner or *Hygienist* has performed his whole duty in merely acting as a "medical" adviser or treater of disease at the bedside of the sick and dying. He should at all times, be a teacher engaged in teaching the people how to live to avoid disease. This means that he should seek to make his services dispensable.

A true science of disease prevention, or of health building can rest upon correct principles only and these were discovered by *Hygienists*. What do these discoveries imply in practice? What principle did they establish in the healing art? Simply obedience to the laws of life. We cannot depart from them without incurring sickness. We cannot live in disobedience thereunto without perpetuating disease. Is there anything so strange, so astonishing in the proposition that the sick, in order to regain health, should obey the laws of life, just as much as should the well to preserve it? And yet, almost the whole world behaves in accordance with the ridiculous and incomprehensible muddle of medical men, that wholesome things are only adapted to the state of health, while unwholesome things are necessary for the conditions of disease.

These principles teach us plainly that a life which secures the greatest amount of bodily and mental vigor, which insures the longest period of earthly existence, which promotes the highest earthly happiness, and gives the utmost ability to do good in the world is only to be realized in the proper use of all things of earth and the abuse of none. Thus the *Hygienic* school supplies the strongest incentive which can be offered men, women and children to be "temperate in all things."

It is much easier to be well than sick. All nature is pledged to the maintenance and recovery of health. Health comes of itself, but we are in great pains to get our diseases. The elements of an unbounded success are wrapped up in the doctrine of health by healthful living. The statement of Dr. H. Lahn that the best medicine in all climates is a natural mode of living, may be changed to read: the best prophylactic in all climates is a natural mode of living.

It is much easier to keep the body in health than it is to restore it to health once it has become impaired. It is much easier to keep from developing bad habits than it is to break these habits after they have become fixed. How much better, then, to study *Hygiene* and use it to preserve health, than to study the intricacies and mysteries of *materia medica* and endeavor to restore health after it has been lost.

Our lives are so out of line with nature and our habits of thinking are in such perfect conformability with our lives, that we rarely conceive of the health and happiness that may be ours by a simple return to a normal mode of living. The ways of nature are not those of convention. We have strayed far from the paths of nature; so far indeed, that the ways of nature seem foreign to us. As a consequence, a "pernicious malady" is spreading among people and individuals, sapping them of physical and mental fiber. Until this malady is checked or remedied there can be no assurance of permanent health. The remedy will not be found in the realm of scientific research nor laboratory experiment. It can be found only when the people give up their unnatural ways and adjust themselves to the ways of nature.

Marvelously simple are all the works of nature; all the operations of her laws. To our perverted instincts and miseducated senses all may be complexity and confusion. The man who is himself in false relations to everything else will pronounce the whole universe to be chaos. The person who is in harmony with all other objects will find order, beauty, happiness everywhere.

Wonderfully plain are all the teachings of the ever-open volume of nature's book. Every page tells us of the laws of life, the conditions of health, the essentials of a better individuality, of a higher personality. All that we call good, and everything we term evil, are equally our guides and teachers. They lead us in the way we should go, or punish us when we are in the way we should not go, and compel us, as it were, to fulfill the design of nature.

Our present health, our earthly happiness, our personal development, our usefulness to others, our influence on the generations yet unborn, depend on the knowledge of a few exceedingly simple conditions, and our observance of them.

These *Hygienists* have endeavored for over a hundred years to teach the people. We have taught that health is the normal condition of the human race. We have explained the way in which it is to be attained and preserved. Thousands have adopted our principles, and, in their lives, demonstrated their truthfulness and utility. But many more thousands there are who have never heard of them, or who have not that thorough understanding of the subjects they involve, which enables them to make, under all the varied circumstances of life the proper application.

It is indeed no small task to eradicate from society the accumulated errors of three thousand years; to convince the people of the utter fallacy of the popular medical system; to explode all of its false philosophy; to clear the ground of the rubbish of ages, and build up a new, a different, an independent medical science and healing art. But it must be done. It will be done.

These principles have a direct bearing upon the morals of the individual and of society. All good men will be better men by living in obedience to physiological law and thus enjoying good health; conversely, a bad man will be a worse man precisely in the ratio that he departs from the laws of his being in his voluntary habits. There is, in our judgment, a natural and determinate relation between internal conditions and outward conduct.

In medicine and religion poisons and penances take the place of truth and righteousness. Physicians profess to have provided man with means of escaping the natural and inevitable consequences of his conduct. Why, therefore, seek to know the right and do it? Why be good when you can buy absolution? Why avoid the causes of disease when you may be immunized against them? Why search for causes when a pill will set everything right? Why avoid injurious practices, when penicillin will erase their consequences? Why live cleanly when vaccines can make unclean living safe? Why behave lawfully when a sermon or a pill can annul the laws of life? Why think of consequences when we can beg, buy, borrow or steal a cure?

The physician, perhaps innocently because by his professional deeds, ignorantly acts as an abetter of vice, and perhaps crime, by professing to show how to escape by medical penance from the consequences of violations of the laws of life. By the mystical contents of his materia medica, by professional legerdemain, he professes to be able to counteract the operations of the laws of nature. He virtually proposes to the weak-minded inducements for violation of the laws of their being. Thus he leads the human race on to its deterioration. The absurdity, even the wickedness, of such a practice is apparent to all who will bestow a little thought upon it. If such things were really possible they would demoralize the race; for they would automatically license us to do wrong.

Teach men that nature's laws can be broken at pleasure, and mended when convenient; that they can violate all the laws of their being, and find immediate advantage or enjoyment in so doing, and then, when the consequences have become very grievous, they can resort to remedies to restore them to their former state of health, and they will do just what the majority of people the world over are led to do by their medical advisers — they will go on living in utter recklessness of nature's laws, incurring all manners of diseases, and employing physicians and "healers" of various kinds to dose away and treat away the inevitable consequences of their reckless follies. These doctrines of the shaman are the most demoralizing doctrines that have ever been entertained by the human mind.

Hygienists assert that, the world's redemption from disease, doctors, and drugs, depends on a practical recognition of the doctrine that nature's laws cannot be violated with impunity; that penalties will not be remitted; that nature has not provided remedies; that if wrong is done, evil consequences will follow; that every poisonous drug, and every unphysiological habit, and every unhealthful act, will make its injurious mark irreparably and forever; that our life, our strength, our health, will be measured exactly by our observance of organic law. This is a statement of a vital truth, the full realization of which, by the people as a whole, will lead inevitably to a revolution in their various modes of living. For the beginning of *Hygienic* wisdom is to "cease to do evil." It will be easy thereafter to "learn to do good."

Health and disease are according to obedience and disobedience. If wrong is done, evil consequences must follow. There are great errors in our habits of life, as evidenced by the great amount of faulty development, sickness and premature dying among us. But we cannot wipe these errors out with drugs, vaccines, serums, gland extracts, and the surgeon's knife. Nor can we ignore the errors of life. To teach that drugs are better than obedience and that the pathological products of animal sacrifices are better than conformity with the laws of life, is to completely demoralize all who accept and believe such doctrines. It is folly to think that consequences can be dosed or vaccinated away. Nature has made no provision to nullify nor destroy her own laws. The only real cure is a return to obedience. Nature does not bribe us to sin by promising us absolution. She does not hold out to us any hope that we may escape the consequences or effects of our unphysiological conduct by resort to any immunizing agent. There is no basis in all nature for the doctrine of immunization. Immunity, were it real, would mean the suspension of the law of cause and effect.

The best, indeed the only, method of promoting individual and public health is to teach people the laws of nature and thus teach them how to preserve their health. Immunization programs are futile and based on the delusion that the law of cause and effect can be annulled. Vaccines and serums are employed as substitutes for right living; they are intended to supplant obedience to the laws of life. Such programs are slaps in the face of law and order. Belief in immunization is a form of delusional insanity.

Obliterate these false doctrines of cure and immunization from medical schools, and books, teach the people the simple truth in relation to the nature of disease, the *modus operandi* of so-called remedies, and the theory of stimulation, and we shall have gone a long way towards the physical regeneration of the people.

Teach this generation the true relations between living and lifeless matter and the next generation will sing the song of a new redemption. Teach men and women to prevent disease by avoiding its causes rather than to attempt to cure it by administering the causes of other diseases and health and happiness will abound everywhere. If the people can be thoroughly indoctrinated with the principles of physiology and *Hygiene,* they will have very little need of physicians; and when they understand the nature of disease and the *modus operandi* of medicines, they will never consent to be poisoned because they are sick.

We are convinced that mankind can be educated in correct principles and trained in right practices so that sickness will cease to trouble us. It is our business to teach people how to prevent disease and not merely how to care for themselves when ill. We are not content to be mere tinkers and patchworkers. We are fully convinced also that the old medical systems and the present trends in medicine have mankind headed in the wrong direction.

I am well aware of the revolutionary character of the principles I have presented. I know that their acceptance by the public will work great changes, not only in the care of the sick and in the prevention of disease, but in many other fields of modern activity, but I am convinced that the physical salvation of our race depends upon their acceptance.

DR. ISAAC JENNINGS ON VITALITY AND DISEASE

The new theory holds that disease is simply a negation of health, a depressed and impaired state of the movements and condition of the system, occasioned immediately or proximately by deficiency of vital power, remotely by the operation of impairing causes. That vital action in man is one and the same under all circumstances; that this vital principle or power is itself under the government of law, a law as fixed and uniform in its mode of operation as the laws of gravitation, or any other natural law; and that consequently, when a perfectly developed and sound human system is amply supplied with this motive principle, there will be a perfect healthy action; and when this power becomes deficient from over draft or excessive use, or when an impediment to its free action is interposed by a damaged state of the instruments of motion, by direct injury, action falters, becomes less efficient, and deviates more or less from the common or usual standard of healthy action, and, by necessary consequence, is followed by a corresponding vitiation of the solids and fluids.

In other, more general and comprehensive language, disease consists,

First, in a damaged state of the system either in vitiation of matter or diminution of force, or both, superinduced by the operation of noxious causes or influences.

This, in part, may or may not be perceptible by human senses. Sometimes individuals are pushed quite to the outer verge of life, without being conscious of it themselves, or giving any intimation of it to the others, and suddenly drop the "mortal coil," when it is not in the power of man to prevent it, and yet no trace of structural derangement or organic defect shall be discoverable on the most extensive and minute post mortem examination.

The quantity of vital power, or force or strength of vitality in store at any time, is not within human ken. In one case it may be near final exhaustion without premonition, and yet sustain all the functions at a high point of healthy action, up to the very moment of total and inevitable cessation; while in another case it will hold out beyond all human calculation, carry the system through astonishing changes, and at length restore it to soundness.

* * *

So strong is the upward tendency of vitality — disposition of present vital derangement, or departure from the highest state of health—that every opportunity, every period of rest, every favorable circumstance, will be improved to repair injuries, and clothe with power, without suffering any sensible demonstration thereof to be made. And this disposition or tendency can never change—turn about and operate in a wrong direction—under any condition of the system, or change of circumstances, any more than the tendency of water to run down hill can change, and dispose rivers to turn back and move up inclined planes.

—*Excerpts taken from a rare pamphlet—"Defense and Appeal" 1847.*

Chapter XI

No. 665. "If we would correctly ascertain how man must live in order to secure the most perfect health and attain to the greatest age of which the human constitution is capable, we must not ransack society to find all the remarkable instances of longevity, and learn the particular habits of those who have attained to old age: —for such a course would only serve to bewilder and perplex us, and lead us to conclude that the whole question is involved in the most entire uncertainty: because we should find health and old age in almost every variety of circumstances in which mankind is placed; and if we were not fully qualified for the severest and most critical investigation of such an intricate subject, we should inevitably misapprehend facts, and thus be led to erroneous conclusions: —but we must study the human constitution with the most rigorous scrutiny of science. —We must analyze the human body to its organic elements, and become thoroughly acquainted with all the elementary tissues which enter into the formation of all its organs, and fully understand the peculiar vital properties of all those tissues and the functional powers of all the organs. We must intimately and accurately know all the conditions on which the peculiar properties of the tissues and powers of the organs depend, and the various causes and circumstances by which those properties and powers are favorably or unfavorably affected. —In short, we must ascertain all the properties and powers which belong to the living animal body, and all the laws of constitution and relation appertaining to the vital economy of the human system. —Here, and only here, can the enlightened and truly scientific physiologist take his stand, and teach those rules of life, by which man may with greatest certainty secure the best health and attain to the greatest longevity of which the human constitution is capable.

"But while the truly scientific physiologist, from his intimate and thorough knowledge of all the properties and powers, and laws of constitution and relation, belonging to the human body, instructs us how to live in order to secure the highest degree of health, and attain to the longest life of which the human constitution is capable, he cannot from this knowledge, tell us what the capabilities of the human constitution are in regard to health and longevity. He can tell us with accuracy and confidence that, such and such are the laws of life—and such and such are the best means by which health may be secured and life prolonged: —but he cannot, from his physiological knowledge, tell us whether a strict obedience to the laws of life, and a correct use of the best means, will prolong our life ten, or a thousand years.

"If therefore, we ask the truly enlightened physiologist, *how* we must live to secure the best health and longest life of which our constitution is capable, — his answer must be drawn purely from the physiological knowledge: —but if we ask him how long the best mode of living will preserve our life, his reply is, "Physiology cannot teach you that. Therefore, now go you out into the world and find the oldest man living and enjoying health.— If after having obeyed his command, we return and say to him, we have found several individuals a hundred years old and all enjoying pretty nearly the same degree of health; yet they are of very different and even of opposite habits, his answer will be that probably each of the individuals you have found has a mixture of good and bad habits, and has lived in a mixture of favorable and unfavorable circumstances, and that, notwithstanding the apparent diversity of habits and circumstances among them, there is probably a pretty nearly equal amount of what is salutary and conservative in the habits and circumstances of each and all. Some of them have erred in one thing and some in another, and some have been correct in one thing and some in another, and therefore the diversity of which you speak is probably more apparent than real, in relation to the true laws of life. Besides, some, with an extraordinarily powerful constitution, may, in the constant violation of the laws of life, reach a hundred years with as much health and vigor, as others who attain to the same period in much better habits and circumstances, but with far less powerful constitutions. All that is proved therefore, by instances of longevity in connection with bad habits and circumstances is that such individuals possess remarkably powerful constitutions, which are able to resist for ninety or a hundred years causes that have in the same time sent hundreds of thousands of their fellow creatures, of feeble constitutions, to an untimely grave; and which, under a correct regimen, would in all probability have sustained life and health a hundred and twenty, and perhaps a hundred and fifty years. —The only use which you can safely make therefore, of the instances of great longevity which you have found," he would say, "is to show how long the human constitution, in the present age of the world and condition of the race, is capable of resisting the causes which induce death: —and if you have found an individual or a number of individuals a hundred years old, it is of little importance to you how they have lived, —the simple fact that they are a hundred years old is all we wish, to prove that the human constitution is now capable of reaching a hundred years." — *Sylvester Graham, 1839.*

IMPAIRED ELIMINATION

Dr. James C. Jackson

Written in 1862

The imperfect performance of the function of depuration is often a chief cause of morbid states of the blood. When we consider the importance of the changes that take place in the lungs; the quantity of carbonaceous fluids constantly discharged through this organ, and of watery vapor, loaded with various impurities, continually exhaled from its surface, and passing out with the expired air; or the abundant perspiration, sensible as well as insensible, constantly issuing from the cutaneous surface, and holding dissolved in it substances which require to be eliminated from the circulation (owing either to their excess or their foreign and hurtful nature); or the varying state of the urinary secretion; or the secretions formed by the liver, the internal surfaces of the bowels, pancreas, etc., out of elements, which, if not combined into these new forms and destined to serve ulterior purposes, would become poisonous to the frame by vitiating the blood.—IT MUST BE EVIDENT, THAT INTERRUPTION OF ANY OF THESE FUNCTIONS, IF NOT COMPENSATED FOR BY THE VICARIOUS INCREASE OR MODIFICATION OF SOME OF THE OTHERS, MUST BE FOLLOWED BY ALTERATIONS OF THE QUANTITY, OF THE QUALITY, AND OF THE RELATIVE PROPORTIONS, OF THE CONSTITUENTS, AND EVEN OF THE VITALITY, OF THIS FLUID. Under the due dominance of the vital energy of the system, and particularly of that influence exerted by the organic nerves on the great secreting viscera and on the whole vascular system, no sooner does any substance which may have been carried into the circulation, or which may have accumulated in it, become injurious, than it is eliminated by the proper action or in the state of its secretions, according to the nature of the substance which affects it. Thus we perceive various substances, and kinds of food, affecting the action and secretions of the kidneys, of the skin, and of the bowels, even in health; certain of their constituents becoming sensible in the halitus of the expired air, in the perspiration, or in the urine, where they come to be transported through the channel of the circulation only. The fetor, etc., of the breath, and the perspiration, etc., of the skin, upon interruptions of the abdominal secretions, indicate also that impuritives have accumulated in the circulation, and that they are being eliminated by means of the lungs and skin. SO LONG AS THE VITAL ENERGY IS SUFFICIENT FOR THE DUE PERFORMANCE AND HARMONY OF THE FUNCTIONS, INJURIOUS MATTERS ACCUMULATE LESS FREQUENTLY, TO THE EXTENT OF VITIATING THE CONSTITUTION OF THE BLOOD: BUT WHEN, FROM ANY CAUSE, THIS ENERGY LANGUISHES, OR IS DEPRESSED BY EXTERNAL AGENTS OR INFLUENCES, AND THE BLOOD IS THEREBY EITHER IMPERFECTLY FORMED, OR ANIMALIZED AND DEPURATED INSUFFICIENTLY, SOME ONE OF ITS ULTIMATE ELEMENTS OR PROXIMATE CONSTITUENTS BECOMES EXCESSIVE, AND THE CHIEF CAUSE OF A DISORDER, WHICH TERMINATES EITHER IN THE REMOVAL OF THE MORBID ACCUMULATION, OR IN A TRAIN OF MORBID ACTION AND ORGANIC LESIONS.

SUNLIGHT

Common observance ought to teach us the value of sunlight, as a factor in health. Whether in the animal or vegetable kingdom, its influence is indispensible to healthful conditions, and therefore, to perfect growth and development. Deprive a plant or flower of sunlight, and immediately it droops and fades; it cannot live without it. Place a vine in a dark cellar, and if there is a window within reach it will incline toward it; and where there is insufficient light it becomes pale and sickly, showing a want of that life-giving element. If suddenly removed from its dark environment, and placed in the strong light and heat of the sun's rays, these may wither and perhaps kill it. Does it follow that sunlight and heat are not food for the plant? On the contrary, it proves that the lack of them has sapped its vitality; that instead of being hardy and well developed in every part, it has become weak and unhealthy.

The same is true of the human plant; by shutting it up in a dark place where the sun's rays seldom or never enter, we impair constitutional vigor and lay the foundation for a wasting disease. Lack of sunlight and pure air are among the leading causes of scrofula, pulmonary tuberculosis and kindred affections; though the decline may be hastened in other ways, as by errors in diet, and insufficient or improper clothing. So important are the sun's rays to life and health, that this great luminary has been called the source of all life, animal and vegetable. It is unquestionably necessary to its highest forms, and also to good health. Moreover, when health is lost or impaired, sunlight is one of the best agents for restoring it. This is particularly true in all those diseases which involve the glands, or the nervous system. In tubercular affections, nothing is so essential to recovery as an abundant supply of pure air and sunlight. The patient should live and exercise in them as much as possible, in order to get well. The sun bath, properly given, is also excellent.

By Dr. Susanna Way Dodds, 1900.

CAUSES OF DISEASE

If good health is the product of right living, sickness or ill health must necessarily result from wrong living. Like causes produce like effects, all through nature; this is as true in the domain of life as it is in physics or mathematics. But the effects that follow obedience and transgression are unlike as possible. The one brings happiness, the other, misery and suffering. If, by the careful observance of the laws of physiology, vital action is well balanced and perfect health secured, we have but to violate these laws in order to produce sickness and death. Life is lengthened and filled with joy by living in accordance with nature's teachings; it is not only shortened but rendered miserable and worthless by pursuing an opposite course.

By Susanna Way Dodds, M. D., 1915.

NATURAL HYGIENE SCIENCE

It cures sick people by removing the cause of sickness.

It removes the disease by removing the necessity for it.

It believes nature is right, and hence does not seek to thwart her operations.

It declares that disease is a natural process of purification, and should not be stopped, but aided.

Its remedies are Nature's health preservatives. Obedience to nature is its greatest panacea. Air, light, food, water, exercise, rest, sleep, etc., in such manner and degree as nature can use are its curatives. Remove the Cause, and the effect will cease, is Hygienic science.

By Robert Walter, M. D., 1894.

NATURAL HYGIENE

Let us get a clear conception of what is meant by the phrase Natural Hygiene. . . . It should be obvious that any hygiene, to be genuine, must be natural. Why, then, not use merely the term Hygiene, as did Graham, Jennings, Alcott, Trall, Densmore, Page, Walter, Oswald, Tilden, etc.? We have adopted the phrase Natural Hygiene to distinguish the employment of forces and substances that have a constitutional relation to the living organism from the employment of measures and processes that are abnormal, anti-vital and which have no normal relation to life. At the time Graham, Trall and their co-workers adopted the phrase the Hygienic System, the medical profession gave no attention to hygiene. Since that time they have created an artificial, anti-vital and spurious hygiene which has made it essential that we employ a phrase that distinguishes our work from theirs. Although Dr. Shelton is probably the first man to recognize the need for this qualifying adjective with which to designate our Hygiene, it was agreed upon by a meeting of Hygienists at the Fourth Annual Convention of the American Natural Hygiene Society - Program.

TOXEMIA
The Universal Cause of all Diseases
By J. H. Tilden, M. D.

WHAT IS DISEASE? The answer to this question is a part of the answer to the question: "What is truth?" Truth is always so simple and commonplace that it is overlooked for the more pretentious seeming which is ever-present in all minds not educated out of reverence and awe for things not understood.

The child-mind shrinks—withdraws—from the awe-inspiring presence of truth; but if it is induced to examine it, familiarity breeds contempt. The ignorant mind is driven away from truth either by a fear-inspiring awe or by the contempt that familiarity without comprehension breeds. The word "truth" is associated with God, infinite, and universe, and is looked upon as beyond the understanding of the finite mind.

The education of man up to date has been of such a character as to cause him to belittle anything within his comprehension and to extol all which he does not understand. The teachings of today are that truth is a part of God, and that God is incomprehensible, hence beyond man's finding out.

This statement regarding our—I might say human—ignorance may be disputed, but the beliefs and teachings of those who will dispute my statement are all the proofs I need for substantiation.

If man is to get anywhere in the line of understanding, he must cease to be inspired into awe by the immensity and supposed incomprehensibleness of God—of the All—and at the same time dispute the divinity of the truth that is within his comprehension. We must accept commonplace facts and recognize them as the units—as cells—out of which God is built, and that, if we know all about a unit of any of the infinities out of which God is built, we have a working hypothesis with which to measure God Himself.

If we learn the truth about the influence of coffee, fear, awe, or anything that stimulates and enervates (produces disease in) our bodies, we have learned a unit of truth which, if we really understand, will give us the key to unlock the whole mystery of disease, its causes and cure.

A true philosophy of healing must rest upon a true interpretation of what disease is, and its cause and cure. Disease *per se* has no existence; it is simply perverted health; and health is a state of being which ranges from comfort to discomfort. When we are comfortable, and enjoy work and recreation, we call this state health; when we have pain, and take no pleasure in work or play, this state we call disease. Health is normal and natural; the opposite is abnormal, and we call it disease.

The old—should-be obsolete—idea that God—Good—has a rival for honor and power in the Devil—Bad—is the foundation of our ethics; and, medically speaking, this idea leads to the erroneous belief in cure.

God, or Nature, stands for everything. There are no antithetical deities or entities. When these facts of experience give way to apparent opposites, it is due to an unfavorable point of view. The real returns when we adjust ourselves amicably to the laws of our being—to nature's requirements.

The cause of disease is any influence that lowers or perverts the normal standard of health.

The study of disease *per se* leads to chaos. Only *knowledge of health*—the study of health—can give a true knowledge of what we call disease.

TOXEMIA, THE UNIVERSAL, BASAL CAUSE OF ALL SO-CALLED DISEASES

The toxin may be autogenerated, or it may be taken into the system from without.

The medical world has been looking for a remedy to cure disease, notwithstanding the obvious fact that nature needs no remedy—she only needs an opportunity to exercise her own prerogative of self-healing.

Only the other day a sick doctor offered a million dollars for a cure for cancer. If he had been philosophically, as well as scientifically, educated, he would not have died believing in the possibility of a cure after nature had passed her eternal fiat of unfitness on any case.

There are no cures for disease. Health, and how to build it and keep it, is the knowledge needed. All the medical hypotheses so far advanced by the profession are largely antithetical and inconsistent, if not wholly out of unison with any synthetic theory of the universe that

— 58 —

has been advanced by scientists, so far as known—except, of course, the Mosaic; and this the leaders in medical science would be loath to acknowledge as their scientific basis, notwithstanding the fact that their pet theory, bacteriology, rests wholly on it, and that without it the germ theory cannot be explained.

For twenty-five years I practiced the science of medicine. During most of that time I did not know why people were sick, why they got well, nor why they died.

When visiting the sick, and treating them in the most approved style, I had no idea of how I should find them at the next call. I did not know if the disease would end soon or late. I did not know if it would take on a severe form, or quickly run its course. I did not know whether or not there would be complications. In fact, I did not know anything that would make me comfortable regarding the outcome of the disease; and, of course, I could not say anything of a real comforting nature to my patients or their friends. I had the usual stock-in-trade subterfuges and little nothings that are worked off on a confiding public by the profession everywhere. Here is one, for example: "If no complications arise, the patient will recover."

Was my experience unique? Was it peculiarly my own? Not by any means. My experience in those days was an exact duplicate of the experiences of the best, as well as the worst, physicians today. I defy the so-called best practitioners of this or any other country to undertake to prove that what I am saying is not true. Not one of the best practitioners can tell from one day to another how his patients will be. Not one can truthfully say that there is not an element in every case that is not known to him, and not knowable. Not one can say with any certainty that the drug he prescribes will have the action he hopes to experience. Not one can tell, after the first twenty-four hours of medication, whether the symptoms presenting themselves are those of disease proper or are due to drugs. Not one can tell after the disease has been under treatment for a day or two, whether his patient is suffering from disease free from drug action, food poisoning, deranged emotions, or mental depression.

To sum up: No doctor, from the professor in college to those in the rear rank, knows anything definite about his patients after the first day's drugging. Every honest doctor will admit that there is an unknown quantity about every case he treats which forces him to guess if asked to give his opinion. This wholesale guesswork is made necessary because the whole scheme of theory and practice is an unorganized mass of theory, science, empiricism and superstititon. Every disease is looked upon as an individuality; each disease—name—has a special germ created to cause it. Nonsense! This is no more the truth than that words are made up of letters independent of the alphabet. As truly as every word must go back to the alphabet for its letter elements, every disease must go back to toxemia, and the causes of toxemia, for its initial elements.

The toxin theory of the healing art is grounded on the TRUTH that TOXEMIA is the basic source of all diseases. So sure and certain is this truth that I do not hesitate to say that it is by far the most satisfactory theory that has been advanced in all the history of medicine. It is a scientific system that covers the whole field of cause and effect—a system that synthesizes with all knowledge, hence a true philosophy.

When this truth first began to force itself upon me, years ago, I was not sure but that there was something wrong with my reasoning. I saw that it would bring me very largely in opposition to every established medical treatment. I held back, and argued with myself—I was afraid that I was developing a self-destructive egomania. I fought to suppress giving open utterance to a belief that would, in all probability, cause me to be hissed at—subject me to the jeers and gibes of the better class of people, both lay and professional.

Little by little I have proved the truth of my theory. I have tried it out daily for the past twenty years. I myself have personally stood the brunt of my experimenting, and have willingly suffered because of it. Every day this trying-out of the theory has convinced me more and more that TOXEMIA IS THE UNIVERSAL CAUSE OF DISEASE.

So simple and so matter-of-fact are all the truths of this toxin theory that it is a surprise that every professional man has not also discovered them. Indeed, the simplicity of it all has caused me to hesitate to write about it; for, strange to say, people generally hate the simple things of life. It has been hard for me to convince myself that there could be so much in so little—so simple—a theory.

The truth is so revolutionary that it will not be adopted at once. The profession is not ready for it; for just now the profession is enthusiastically occupied with the germ theory—a theory which declares that a specific germ causes a specific disease; a theory which in time must die out, the same as every other false theory.

My theories have received but little attention. A few, a very few, physicians know what I stand for. Those few, however, are enthusiastic, and have proved to their own satisfaction that the theory has a universal application.

I have been urged by many to define my theory and practice. I really have defined it thousands of times in the past ten years—not in any formal statement, but in my writings—in such a way that any professional mind should have had no trouble in interpreting it, if it had given my writings the attention a student mind should. Indeed, any professional mind should have read this theory in almost every number of my periodical; for I have not attempted to disguise it at any time, but, on the contrary, have made it tantalizingly plain to any but prejudiced minds.

Professional minds are supposed to be trained into a power of discrimination that enables them to sense truth in anything. But it appears that the principal training today is into accepting authority without question.

I should not be accused of rushing into print, and handing out an immature theory to the public; for I have been proving it for years.

To define just what is meant by toxemia, I will say: Toxemia means poisoned by toxin taken into the body, or by one's own waste products —retained metabolic waste—brought about by inefficient elimination; and faulty elimination is caused by enervation—a weakened state of the body—lost resistance.

The body is strong or weak, as the case may be, depending entirely upon whether the nerve energy is strong or weak. And it should be remembered that the functions of the body are carried out well or badly according to the amount of energy generated.

It should be known that without nerve energy not an organ of the body—a gland or muscle—can perform its function. This being true, reason declares that there must be a limit to the supply of this energy, and that each organism requires a specific amount. The amount, under normal conditions, it is safe to assume, is just what is necessary to do the work of the organism with the least amount of wear and tear.

For the human body to function normally—for the physiological processes to be carried on in an ideal way—just the proper amount of nerve energy must be generated. This means that waste and repair are adjusted to ordinary needs, and that for these needs sufficient energy is generated to carry on the work. But no provision can be made for the supply of more energy for extraordinary demands, such as are experienced in civilized life. Work, worry, and the pleasure-seeking peculiar to civilization draw heavily on the capital stock of nerve energy. The consequence is that everyone is in a more or less enervated state. This weakened state—this state of used-up nerve energy—shows itself in imperfect elimination. The inability of the organism to rid itself of waste products brings on *Autotoxemia.* That this is universal cannot be successfully disputed, for *it is impossible to find one human being, in the ordinary walks of life, free from self-poisoning.* If enervation is the cause of *Autotoxemia,* then why is not enervation the cause of all diseases? Because weakness is not sickness. Poison is the only sickness *per se.* Man can be enervated, yet not sick; but he cannot be poisoned —sick—without being enervated.

As has been stated continuously in my writings for the past dozen years, the habits of overeating, overclothing, and excesses of all kinds use up nerve energy. When the nerve supply is not equal to the demands of the body, organic functioning is impaired, resulting in the retention of waste products. This produces *Toxemia.*

There is a heavy draft on nerve supply caused by our modern manner of living, and it is not strange that all active people are more or less enervated. Enervation cannot be enduring without developing self-poisoning, because an enervated body cannot and will not eliminate the waste products as it should.

"The large percentage of men refused by the army physicians because of physical defects has 'shocked' the nation." Why? Echo answers, "Why?" Because the truth of toxemia is ignored or not understood.

The longer toxemia exists, the less nerve energy or resistance there is. Hence those with the least resistance are the first to go down under strain, let that be physical exertion, excitement, self-abuse in overindulgence of the appetites or passions, weather conditions, or any influence requiring nerve energy to resist.

This theory, and this theory alone, gives a satisfactory reason for epidemic influences. To maintain animal life in health and vigor, variety is necessary and monotony must be avoided. If there is one thing more striking than another in all natural phenomena, it is change. On the world-stage, actors and scenery change rapidly. Action is life; inactivity is death.

Single ideas evolve monomaniacs. The continuous sowing of one variety of farm products ruins the soil; water not in motion becomes stagnant.

When weather conditions are monotonous—when heat, cold, wet, or dry is continued beyond a given time—the effect on animal life is enervating and conducive to disease. This is what should be recognized as the epidemic influence. When it exists, all the people living in such section of country are more or less affected by it. Those who are already enervated to the point of a breakdown, from bad habits and unwholesome domestic and civic environments, become victims of the epidemic influence.

Localities in which the people are already enervated to the collapsing point, because of their lack of cleanliness, suffer more than other localities that give intelligent attention to cleanliness.

FEAR IS AN ALLY OF EPIDEMIC INFLUENCE

Nothing is so depressing and nerve-annihilating as fear. That is why so many succumb to epidemic influences. Fear, added to the epidemic influence, kills many who would not come down from the epidemic influence without it. Fear kills as many in the every-day diseases as any other influence. Those who go through epidemics without contracting the disease are those who are not badly toxemic and who are devoid of fear.

True enlightenment is one of the most potent remedial influences. An enlightenment that teaches man to believe in disease being inevitable is disease-provoking. Fear is a child of ignorance. Intelligence banishes fear; hence intelligence is one of the greatest conservators of nerve energy. When the people are intelligent enough to banish fear of disease —when they understand that the more they conserve their nerve energy by poise, and by avoiding unnecessary expenditure of nerve force, the healthier they will be—disease generally will be stamped out. When people are intelligent enough to give themselves self-protection, they will know the importance of perfect personal cleanliness, and civic cleanliness and drainage; after which health will be the rule, and not the exception, as we now see it. It is as necessary that man's systemic drainage be in perfect working order as it is that his civic drainage be perfect. Flushing is all right in the civic system, but in man's system it has proved a failure.

Chronic toxemia is the unknown element that forms the basis of all chronic diseases. When this constant element is recognized and reckoned with in planning a treatment for any disease, the element of uncertainty that makes guesswork neecssary, and such a huge nightmare of *all healing systems,* will pass away, and certainty, with its restfulness to doctor, patient, and friends, will be experienced.

The idea that the cause of disease must be an entity has dominated the medical mind from the earliest time. It is false. *Disease is simply health pushed aside by influences that lower life's standard. Health is the normal state of the body, and all the body's energies are directed to its maintenance.*

When toxemia is accepted as the underlying principle which makes all diseases kin, doctors can proceed in the treatment of all diseases with a certainty and confidence never before experienced by physicians. Uncertainty will be a thing of the past.

When a doctor knows that the underlying constitutional derangement of Bright's disease, tuberculosis, or cancer, is one and the same thing, he can go to work with a knowledge and a confidence unknown to so-called scientific medicine. Then there will be no more excuse for sectarianism in medicine; for all theories of cure must come to one universal cause. And when all recognize one cause, there can be no excuse for such a conglomeration of therapeutic measures as is advocated today by the various systems of healing, and which amounts to a stupendous plan of palliation.

What brings on toxemia? Any habit or social custom that uses up nerve energy and brings on enervation. Enervation must always act in one way; namely, to check elimination. This causes waste products to be pent up in the organism. And when this condition is present, we have, first, last, and all the time, TOXEMIA. This is so self-evident that the wonder is that physicians generally have not recognized it long ago. Why I recognized this greatest of medical truths I cannot tell, unless it was that I had been forced from one theory to another in my endeavor to find a rational excuse for the universal uncertainty which all thinking physicians must have experienced, in trying to account for the apparently eccentric character of diseases.

MY THEORY AND PRACTICE OF THE HEALING ART ARE ACCORDING TO THE TRUTHS HEREIN ADVANCED

Does the toxin theory work out in practice? It certainly does. If it did not, I should have starved long ago. My practice today is largely confined to so-called incurable diseases. As I have often said, few come to me who can find relief anywhere else; for my prescriptions consist of proscriptions—all habits and styles of living that bring on enervation must be given up. It is impossible to cure any disease unless the cause is recognized and removed; and the cause is anything in the life of the patient that uses up energy. No one should be so blinded by prejudice or preconceptions as to be unable to see the truth of this; for it is so self-evident and obvious that *he who runs should read.*

In acute diseases we see nature making her most profound efforts to get rid of poison. There is a class of diseases known as ptomaine poisoning, which is brought on from eating food that is undergoing decomposition. This poisoning may take place in those with large resistance, where the amount ingested is great. It is possible to have so large an amount taken into the system as to kill outright. But barring such extremes, those who are affected greatly with only a moderate amount of poison are those whose resistance has been broken down by chronic toxin poisoning—by chronic toxemia—from gastro-intestinal decomposition. At first, nature builds a large toleration for toxins; but when resistance is lost, then intolerance sets in, and unless the toxin habit is overcome, organic disintegration ends the struggle.

Chronic Toxemic Subjects, on account of having less resistance, are susceptible to the action of accustomed stimulants. Indeed, when these subjects indulge beyond their digestive capacity, they are often poisoned by having the food they eat decompose. This is auto-infection—self-poisoning.

Typhoid fever, pneumonia, appendicitis, and other diseases of a so-called infectious character are strictly cases of auto-infection. The toxemic subject has so little resistance that, when his digestion is crowded beyond its reduced capacity, decomposition takes place. This, if not discovered and corrected by withholding food, will start a morbid process which will develop a disease of the character of those named above. The surest correction is to stop all food and give water only. When this is done, the morbid process fails to develop typically. Hence, what becomes of the specific cause?

It is said that a special germ causes typhoid, and another special germ causes pneumonia. It can be proved that the subjects of both these diseases have autotoxemia, established by wrong life, to such a degree that their digestions are impaired, and decomposition is going on in the intestines, adding a septic poison to the toxemic. When the decomposition is great, there is a high temperature, which is "necessary to burn up the toxin debris in the blood;" and if the treatment is not death-dealing, these cases will get well. After which, if the individual understands what has taken place in his organism, he can so order his life that another such house-cleaning will not be necessary.

Those who wish to be victimized by false reasoning and sophistry, and who wish to pin their faith to the germ theory and cure of disease, may do so, of course; but there is a drugless, serumless, and surgeryless plan that means less sickness, fewer deformities and mutilations, and decidedly fewer deaths.

Germs furnish the ferment necessary to further elimination; but this is a friendly, rather than a hostile act.

Acute fevers indicate that there has been a sudden absorption of unaccustomed poison, or a sudden absorption of an unusual quantity of an accustomed poison. High fever marks the profoundness of the nervous shock. Where the nervous system is profoundly affected, not infrequently, skin radiation is suspended, and breathing impeded, causing the heat of the body to run up several degrees. Medical science declares that the high grade of fever means the burning-up of disease-producing debris. But this is not logical, hence not believable; for the longer the high grade of fever lasts, the more accumulation there will be of waste products, which are carried out of the body as soon as the nervous system reacts, and secretions and excretions are reestablished. Feeding, or the daily intake of food, keeps a fever burning and waste products accumulating until death relieves the sufferer.

I have seen the temperature in a convalescent run up from normal to 103 degrees, and the pulse go from 80 to 120, within an hour after an imprudent meal that caused acidity; and I have seen such temperature and pulse reduced in thirty minutes to nearly normal by administering twenty to thirty grains of baking-soda, which neutralized the fermentation and relieved the irritation of the nervous system. A stomach lavage would be a more ideal relief. I have seen the temperature of the body and the pulse lowered almost instantly by opening a pent-up pus cavity, or by washing out a septic wound or uterus.

Fever means nerve irritation and depression sufficient to disorganize normal coordination for the time being, cutting off surface radiation. When the nervous system becomes accustomed to toxemia and septic poisoning, acute symptoms subside, and then we have an insidious arthritis, endocarditis, or other chronic disease.

Pent-up secretions, excretions, septic matter or pus cause enough nervous irritation to bring on elevation of temperature and acceleration of pulse; but in time the reactive forces of nature become so blunted that acute symptoms no longer obtain.

The organism may be so abused and enervated that there is no power left for a reaction sufficient to get rid of sepsis or toxemia. Then it is that we have chronic disease—chronic toxemia—with a giving-way of one or more organs of the body. The most vulnerable organ or organs give way. Thus we may have tuberculosis, bronchitis, Bright's disease, colitis, gastritis, or disease of any other organ. The treatment, first, last, and all the time, must be with a view to getting rid of the toxemia. This consists in correcting whatever habits of life are producing enervation, and then gradually building up a normal digestion, assimilation, and elimination. No treatment can be farther from the purpose than the plan advocated by *modern medical science;* namely, giving drugs for relief, which further inhibit elimination, and feeding beyond digestive and eliminative capacity.

We are taught by the very latest development in medical science that germs cause disease. This is untenable to the analytical-minded physician, because, if germs are not omnipresent, their evolvement is imminent, and waits only upon the coalition of the proper environment and elements necessary for their genesis. If the former—if omnipresent—they are not specific at all times. Then to what do they owe their specificity?

The best works on bacteriology declare that all the germs of a supposedly specific character are often found in people who have not had the disease which they—the germs—are supposed to create. Why? Is it not reasonable to assume that their pathological activity waits for a favorable habitat for their toxic transformation and rapid propagation; in other words, that they do not evolve specificity until needed as scavengers? If this is not true, why do they subside and lose their specificity as soon as the pathological habitat is broken up?

It is said that a specific serum has been discovered for infantile paralysis and meningitis. This is a delusion that will be outgrown in time. How can a specific be found for a disease that depends upon a common, primary, universal element—toxemia—either auto- or extra-developed—combined with an exciting cause of a special or peculiar character, such as continuously dry, hot, cold, or moist weather—weather monotony that continues until human beings are enervated and prostrated?

It is impossible to have a specific remedy for a disease that depends upon many diverse elements. There can be no specific remedy any more than there can be a specific cause.

Children who take meningitis, or any of the other so-called contagious diseases, must be autotoxemic from improper food and improper care of the body; and, to bring about an epidemic, there must be an atmospheric state—domestic, civic, or general—that is favorable to intensifying their already large stock of enervation.

Diagnosing, according to *modern medical science,* is so fraught with the element of uncertainty that no reliance can be placed upon it. The specialist is so limited in his knowledge of the philosophy of health and disease that he becomes deluded on the subject; and this delusion often causes him to see meningitis, appendicitis, ovaritis—or any disease that happens to be the subject of his specialty—in every case brought to him. As a matter of fact, most attacks of disease of any and all kinds get well whether treated or not. This fact enables the physician to report a great success for his treatment. Is this an exaggeration? I wish it were.

How about the appendicitis delusion? Nine-tenths of all cases reported are not appendicitis. One case out of twenty diagnosed tumor of the brain may possibly be a correct diagnosis.

Fibroid tumors are credited or said to be the cause of thousands of symptoms. But this statement is refuted by the truth that as soon as improper eating is corrected the patient is relieved and her symptoms disappear, never to return, in spite of the tumor, unless she returns to bad living habits.

When I refer to these delusions leading to mistakes in diagnosis, I do not have in mind the weak members of the profession. I refer only to the best men in it; for the theory and practice of medicine, as practiced today, make fools of the best men in it. No man can be wise enough to steer clear of these professional shoals, so long as he is guided by the science of cause as taught today.

THE ADVANTAGE OF THE IDEA THAT TOXEMIA
IS THE GENERAL CAUSE

What advantage has the toxemic theory over the plan recognized and accepted by the profession of state and nation—namely, the germ theory? The advantage of certainty. It has the advantage that the physician practicing the toxin theory need not live in a constant state of uncertainty about what will become of his patient.

When a child shows symptoms of high fever and vomiting, what is the disease? It may be the beginning of gastritis, scarlet fever, diphtheria, meningitis, infantile paralysis, or some other disease. The treatment, according to my plan, may be positive; there need be no waiting for developments, no guessing, no mistakes. What is done should be the correct treatment for any disease, named or not named; namely, get rid of the causes of the toxemia and the exciting causes, whatever they are. Wash out the bowels—for they are a source of infection, or there would not be fever; then give a hot bath of sufficient duration to furnish complete relief from any pain. When discomfort returns, give another bath. Use an enema every day, and twice daily if symptoms demand. Provide plenty of fresh air and water, and keep the patient quiet. See to it that nothing but water goes into the stomach until the fever and discomfort are entirely overcome; then give very light food at first.

But doctors will say: "Suppose it is a case of diphtheria? Antitoxin should be used, for it is specific!" This will some day be proved a delusion. Remember that this child would not be sick if it were not toxemic, which has reduced its resistanec and made it susceptible to disease-producing influences. Let the local manifestations be what they may, the basic cause is always the same—toxemia plus septic infection; and if this state is not added to by improper treatment—a treatment that still further enervates—the disease will be thrown off quickly. Food adds to the disease. And if food adds to the disease, so will drugs and antitoxins. The disease is *toxin poisoning,* which will soon spend its force if not fed by food or drugs. There is nothing to do *that should be done,* except what I have suggested. If nature is overwhelmed by the poisons—auto- or extra-generated, plus the antitoxin—the patient will die. If the patient gets well when handicapped by food, drugs or antitoxin, it would get well more readily without such interference.

Nature cures, if causes are removed before the vitality is overcome. Any enervating influence—even stimulating treatment—adds to cause.

Those who would go farther into the application of the toxin theory should read my book, *Impaired Health.*

THE UNITY AND SIMPLICITY OF DISEASE

Copyright 1924 by G. R. Clements

Hugo, Oklahoma

... *"If one should maintain his blood in absolute purity, disease would be virtually impossible. The blood is the (life of the flesh) You're what you are, through the influence of the blood that circulates throughout your body."* (Bernarr Macfadden, *Vitality Supreme*, p. 179).

The Universe is a unit. It is the effect of one cause (God). As the whole is made up of the parts, we are for this reason justified in assuming that the whole was produced as the parts are produced. It is inconceivable that there is one order of work for the whole, with a contrary order for the parts. And if the Universe is under the control of one **Law** (Unity of Spirit ... One body and one Spirit—Eph. 4:3,4), how could some parts of it be under the control of some other law?

The body, likewise, is a unit, and it the effect of one cause. Also, the whole is made up of the parts, and the whole was produced as the parts are produced. The same order of work that rules the whole, also rules the parts. Conversely, the same order of work that rules parts of the body, so small that they cannot be seen. is the same order that rules the whole.

Holding this fact before us as our guiding light, we shall proceed to state the primary cause of all disease, and explain the problem so clearly, that anyone of common intelligence can easily understand it. Those accepting "as their doctrines the precepts of men" *(Matt. 15:9)*, may reject this truth because of its sublime simplicity; but we as believers in the Word of God, and not in the tradition of men, should remember that the deepest truths ever expounded have been the simplest and most readily comprehended. There are no exceptions in Nature; therefore the truth as to disease is no exception to the rule of natural simplicity, regardless of all existing complexity and mystery, invented by the greed of gold for its own base ends, now surrounding disease.

The primary cause of disease is nothing more nor less than the (1) wrong use of things supplied by Nature—violation of the Law of God. Since effect follows cause as night follows day, we find the primary effect of the primary cause to be (2) enervation (lowered vital resistance), and toxemia (poison in the blood)—these being the first stages of all bodily disorders. Some authors, who fail to go back to fundamentals for their first principles, mistake the primary effect for the primary cause, and then divide on the question, — one side holding that Toxemia is the primary cause; and the other, that Enervation is. As we shall see, both opinions are erroneous; for the primary cause of disease is not found in the flesh.

It is strange that "science" should seek for the cause of disease nowhere but within the body, and for "cures" nowhere but without, when the real situation is just the reverse. The primary cause of disease is found without; and the only "cure" in the Universe is the curative power of and within the living organism. It was just as sensible to search in the stone for the cause that brings it back to earth, when hurled into the air, or in the rain-drops for the cause of their descent from the clouds, as to search within the body for the cause of disease. Certainly, the study of dead men, and of animals under vivisection, will never reveal the cause of disease; for the cause is invisible, and is not within the body. In fact, all causes are invisible. Newton never saw the Power of Gravitation. He learned of its existence through its effects. Effects only are all that we ever see. Enervation-toxemia is merely the (2) primary effect, while the (1) primary cause, as we have stated, is (1) the violation of the Law of Life.

Having stated the (1) primary cause, and the (2) primary effect, we next ask, what is the (3) secondary cause? In a word, it is the reaction of the body to the internal danger (enervation-toxemia, produced by the (1) violation of law. The violation of the Law of Life invariably produces dangerous internal conditions; and from such conditions the body recoils by instinct, just as a man himself recoils by nature from external danger. The instinctive recoil arises from the spontaneous action of the Great Invisible Force within, which guides and guards the living organism forever and eternally.

We have now come to the (4) secondary effect. Here lies the very crux of the whole matter. Secondary effects have been treated as demons and diseases since the birth of therapeutics, without any knowledge of their underlying and mystifying cause. Today, legions of learned men, termed "scientists," are earnestly engaged in extensive research work, endeavoring to solve the unknown cause of these secondary effects (disease), and learn how to treat, "cure," and prevent them. Drugs, serums, and knives have been and now are the agents used in the attempt to drive these secondary effects from the body, and thus "cure" the "disease." Vaccination and innoculation are practiced to prevent these secondary effects from "attacking healthy bodies." But all efforts have failed and must continue to fail, because the theory is wrong. Due to its vital importance, we shall give the secondary effects by a concrete example.

A man meets an enemy. The man is healthy; his body is normal. The enemy he subdues and conquers after a most strenuous struggle, which leaves him panting for breath, with violent pulsation of the heart, covered with perspiration, without appetite, and weak and exhausted. The additional strength was supplied for the struggle by a general acceleration of all the functions of the body to meet the emergency. The shock of the struggle may be so severe, and the man's strength so depleted, that he becomes unconscious soon after it ends, and is compelled by weakness and exhaustion to lie in bed for several days. However, he soon recovers his former state of health without "treatment" or "medicine" of any sort.

Here is the (4) secondary effect of the body's reaction to threatened danger. The quickening of the functions, being an abnormal state created to counteract an abnormal condition, is followed by a period of weakness and exhaustion, in accordance with the law that "action and reaction are equal, but opposite." We can correctly say that the man, hale, hearty, strong, and vigorous when he met the enemy, is "diseased" ere the battle barely begins; for the abnormal functions (reactions) here noted, are similar indeed to those termed and treated as "disease."

We observe that the (4) secondary effect of the body's reaction to danger within, is similar to that of the body's reaction to danger without —rapid respiration, violent pulsation, profuse perspiration, and a general acceleration of all the functions. However, there is this difference: The danger within arises from an excess of toxins and foreign matter that are corrupting the body; and since the reaction has for its sole purpose the elimination of the destructive internal elements, in the various symptom complexes of vomiting, diarrhea, diphtheria, fevers, pneumonia, smallpox, and other so-called acute diseases, we have and observe the surface indications of this elimination.

As the body concentrates its vital forces for the struggle against the internal danger, a feeling of weakness and fatigue may be noticed. The blood may recede from the surface, and the patient experience a "chill" as a result. When all is in readiness, and not before, a vigorous reaction sets in. The heart begins a violent throbbing that sends the blood rushing in torrents to all parts of the body, and consequently increases the temperature.

The blood is the marvelous stream that turns the wheels of life. As its flow quickens, there is a spontaneous and a simultaneous quickening of the function of all the organs. For the body, as we have said, is a unit, and all parts, under one law, work together, and in perfect harmony with the whole. Therefore, the faster the blood flows, the more intense becomes the action of the Vital Force, and the more powerful is the repulsion and expulsion of all dangerous toxins, morbid matter and waste that are clogging the cells, tissues, and capillaries. Accordingly, the general speeding up of the eliminative organs by the pumping heart and the rushing blood, is indicative of the greatest cleansing and purifying process of which the living organism is capable. The accompanying symptom complexes of "disease," such as vomiting, diarrhea, diphtheria, pneumonia, fevers, smallpox, etc., signify nothing but the various methods adopted by the body for use in purging itself of the dangerous toxins and foreign matter within.

That so-called disease is merely the (4) effects of the body's reaction to dangerous internal elements has been known and understood for ages by a few level-headed, clear-sighted physicians, and is explained in the works of Thomas Sydenham, a master medical man, known as the English Hippocrates. In Vol. 1, p. 29, edition of the Sydenham Society, 1848, we find the following definition of "acute disease" in general:

"A disease, however much its cause may be adverse to the human body, is nothing more than an effort of Nature, who strains with might and main to restore the health of the patient, by the elimination of the morbific matter."

Three-quarters of a century later, Henry Lindlahr, M.D., voiced the same doctrine in these words:

"Every acute disease is the result of a cleansing and healing effort of Nature (p. 55) . . . All acute diseases are uniform in their causes, their purpose, and, if conditions are favorable, uniform also in their progressive development . . ." (*Nature Cure,* 20th Edition, 1922.)

When the nervous system and the reactive forces become adjusted to the pent-up poisons, there is a state of chronic poisoning, wherein the acute symptoms subside, and some chronic ailment is established, which may be some time in progressing to a distressingly noticeable stage. Or, the organism may be so abused and enervated by "scientific treatment," that a reaction sufficient in power to cast off the poisons, is impossible because of a lack of vitality. Then we also have a chronic condition of some sore, such as Bright's Disease, diabetes, cancer, tuberculosis, stomach, liver, or heart trouble, rheumatism, etc. Dr. Lindlahr explains "chronic diseases," as follows:

"To check and suppress acute diseases . . . means to suppress Nature's purifying and healing efforts, to bring about fatal complications, and to change the acute, constructive reactions into chronic disease conditions." (p. 77.)

Going back to our man, we observe that he became "diseased" because during his struggle with the enemy, there was a general speeding up of the function of the body for a specific purpose. When the battle began, and cardiac and respiratory action was accelerated, in an earnest effort to supply the additional strength required in the struggle to subdue the foe, suppose that some "scientist," believing that Nature becomes undependable at times, had stopped the fight, at various intervals, long enough to inject into the man's body some drug and serum poisons, that would bring the functions back to normal by stunning the nervous system and retarding the action of all the various organs? Would this help or hinder the man in the struggle? Would it increase or decrease his strength and vitality? Common sense teaches that it would hinder the man and vastly decrease his strength and vitality, for the procedure is contrary to the functions of the body.

In order to better illustrate our point, we shall say that this is done; for few patients ever pass through illness without being the subject of such "scientific treatment." The body must continue the struggle, for the internal foe (poison) will not depart of its own accord. It must be thrown out by force. So after the interruption for the first injection of drugs and serums, the battle is resumed, somewhat slowly at first on the part of the body, but with increasing vigor as the body recovers from the stunning effect of the drugs and serums.

The battle is soon in full blast again, with the functions of the body running high, in order to supply the requisite strength to carry on the combat to a successful conclusion. The "scientific treatment" is again administered to slow down the functions. This time the body experiences more difficulty to recover from the effect than it did the first time. But it gradually recovers sufficiently to quicken its functions, in a last desperate attempt to supply the strength needed to cast out the foe. And once more is the "scientific treatment" administered to slow down the functions.

The body, we observe, is struggling against two enemies: the physician without and his poisons within, and the original poisons within, which the body endeavored to eliminate by accelerating its functions. Each time that the body was making progress in its work, it received a serious shock at the hands of the physician; and each time this shock occurred, it decreased the body's vitality.

Every living organism is self-operating, self-adjusting, self-repairing, self-preserving and self-curing, and so constituted and formed that each and every function, from birth till death, tends towards health alone, and never towards "disease." By virtue of this, the body will not only maintain itself in health throughout its existence, but will even restore itself to normality when any violation of the Law of Life has created conditions that are incompatible with its harmonious existence: provided the opportunity be given, and the shock induced by the destructive agent be not too severe.

The mal-treatment by "science" here illustrated, was continued until the body was so weakened, that it was at last unable to recover and react because of the gross interference with its functions, and it slowly succumbs—but not to the power of the enemy, for the enemy it would have readily subdued had it not been hampered in its effort. But it succumbs to the power of the poisons administered by the "scientific", misguided physician, who would have the body function as he wants it, and not as Nature would have it.

More harmful and dangerous, and more difficult to eliminate than the different kinds of systematic poisons, originating within the body, are the drugs and serum poisons administered to "cure disease." Every drugless practitioner knows from experience that it is harder to restore a patient who has been under the treatment of an orthodox medical man, and had his body filled with drug and serum poisons, than one who has been under the treatment of none. Dr. Ralph M. Crane, an Osteopath of New York, says that during the winter of 1918 he treated 650 cases of flu-pneumonia, and never lost one; and that in the winter of 1922-23 he treated 125 cases of pneumonia and lost not one. He observed:

"I have never lost one of my own cases, and most of these which come to me after they have been under the care of medical doctors, I can save, with one exception—I cannot do much for patients who have been dosed with morphine, a common practice, I am sorry to say. There is no breaking down through the morphine, even by osteopathy. That drug apparently paralyzes every recuperative faculty a patient possesses."

Knowing that the body is a unit, we know that the law which governs the whole, governs every part. When any part shows signs of sickness, such as throbbing heart, rapid respiration, rising temperature, and so on (which medical men term and treat as disease), we should know that the whole is affected. More than this, we should know that the cause of the visible signs of sickness is merely the (4) secondary effects of the (3) body's reaction to an (2) internal danger, the primary cause of which is (1) violation of law; and that the reaction has for its sole purpose the purging of the body, by its cleansing forces, of the systemic poisons which constitute the dangerous element. This being an abnormal condition, abnormal strength is required, which can be supplied by abnormal function alone, and not by drug and serum poisons that are devoid of life and power of action, and dangerous even to healthy bodies.

Every schoolboy knows that in running, jumping, or in performing any strenuous exercise, additional strength must be furnished for the occasion, and that this is done by the heart, the lungs, and the other organs, vigorously quickening their normal function. Should we interfere with this perfect process of Nature, by slowing down the vital functions with poisons that stun and paralyze the nervous system? Can we safely enforce an arbitrary law as this upon the living organism, in direct violation of its own constitution?

There is reason and purpose in every function of the body. All its functions are perfect, and are designed to accomplish specific results. These results have for their object the improvement of the organism. To "treat" the affected parts—the parts that exhibit the symptoms of "disease"—is to ignore the purpose of the body, to thwart its efforts, and to force upon it an inimical condition that it was striving to cast off. Because we do not understand the body, or its function, or the purpose of its function, does not license any of us, not even "scientists," to assault and attack the body, or any of its parts or functions, with drugs, serums, and knives. To do so must lead only to permanent injury.

We now summarize the cause of disease as follows:

1—Primary cause: violation of the Law of Life.

2—Primary effect: toxemia-enervation.

3—Secondary cause: the body's reaction to the internal danger.

4—Secondary effect: symptom complexes called diseases.

(1) Violation of the Law of Life produces enervation-toxemia; (2) enervation-toxemia threatens the body's harmonious existence; (3) the body reacts to the threatening danger; and (4) the effect of this reaction is exhibited at the surface in symptom complexes termed diseases, of which more than 400 have been named by diagnosticians. To "treat" any "disease" means to "treat" nothing but the effects of the body's reaction to the dangerous internal condition that threatens its destruction, and such course hinders Nature's work.

All substances which, when introduced into the body, either by cutaneous injection or absorption, by respiration or by ingestion, cannot be utilized as food by the body economy, are poisonous thereto. Poisons always force the body to act in self-defense. If the kind and quantity of poison be insufficient to produce instant death, it produces death by degrees by establishing a condition of chronic poisoning (so-called immunity)—a danger to which the body adjusts itself only when it cannot control nor destroy the same. This is observed in the use of tobacco, when the vital resistance must first be subdued, by persistence in the practice, before the body will submit to the poison. In the finale, the destructive agent, which the body was unable to control or destroy, and to which it was forced to yield after its resisting-power was weakened, will compel the body to destroy itself by forcing it continually to act in self-defense, against the ever-present danger, until its Vital Force is exhausted, resulting in a collapse of the nervous system that ultimately brings death.

Every rational person knows that exhaustion kills, even though the body be, in every particular, healthy and vigorous. Twenty-five centuries ago, when the Greeks won the great victory of Marathon, the messenger who brought the news to Athens, ran the entire distance on foot, more than 26 miles, then fell dead from exhaustion as he delivered his message. The machinery of the body functioned so violently and so long, to meet the extraordinary demand made on it, that it simply collapsed from the exhaustive strain.

Diabetes mellitus is a chronically poisoned state of the body, in which the most marked symptom is an excessive amount of saccharine matter and albumin in the urine. All cases of diabetes are benefitted by nothing more than an absolute fast of several days. A diet of uncooked fruits, greens, and vegetables, following the fast, often "cures" the most malignant cases. Why do we suggest uncooked fruits, greens, and vegetables, following the fast? Because no animal, save man, attempts to subsist on "cooked" food; and God has made no exception to law in favor of man in food preparation, or in any other particular. Consequently, here is the (1) primary cause (violation of law) responsible for the chronic poisoning, of which diabetes is one of the many (4) secondary effects. The self-curative power of the body corrects the effect when a chance is given by a removal of the cause; but the effect will return if the cause is resumed.

The (1) primary cause (violation of law) of diabetes is without the body, and is known only by its effect (diabetes) within. Medical men search within for the cause, discover the effect, call that the cause, and Fred Banting "discovers" insulin to "cure" the effect, mistaken for cause, while the cause (violation of law), unnoticed and untouched, remains to continue its deadly work, regardless of all "medical cures"; and Dr. Banting is hailed as the "medical wizard" of the age, and showered with dignities and riches.

In due time, the cause sends the sufferer to an early grave, and weeping friends are evasively told that they waited too long before seeking the services of a "specialist." A profession that forever fails, yet is able by plausible excuses to conceal the cause of its failure, can persuade the gullible public into believing that it is a success, by skillfully shifting the responsibility for its failure to the shoulders of the credulous ones whom it serves and deceives. It requires super-education to enable a deceiver to misrepresent facts so cunningly as to exonerate himself in the eyes of his trustful patients and patrons. "The serpent was more subtile than any beast of the field which God had made."

As surely as every word must go back to the alphabet for its letter-element, just as surely must every "disease" go back to a violation of the Law of Life for its primary cause. And since the secondary cause of "disease" comes from the body's reaction to the dangerous internal condition, we know that every "acute disease" is nothing more or less than the effect of a vigorous effort of the body to protect itself against injurious agents. In other words, that it is purely a curative process in itself, being the normal reaction of the living organism to its environment, and conducted under the guidance of an Infinite Wisdom and Power, that tolerates no interference from human hands, even though offered in a spirit of helpfulness. These vital facts, for facts they are, cannot be reiterated too frequently, nor urged too strongly.

Another point that cannot be too often repeated is this: The signs and symptoms manifested by the body in so-called disease, are not due to the action of the internal poison, in an effort to destroy the organism: for dead matter, being devoid of life, is *ipso facto* devoid of any power of action. Those symptoms, as we have said, are purely the secondary effects of the body's reaction to the internal danger; and when we "treat disease," we simply counteract and suppress the outward signs of the body's efforts to protect itself. There being no such thing as "disease," there can be nothing to treat; and when we do "treat disease," there is nothing accomplished but the counteraction and suppression of the body's natural action of self-protection.

The same is true of all so-called remedies. Drugs and serums do not and cannot act on the body. They are dead matter and dead matter is powerless to act. As Dr. Walter observes:

". . . If drugs are the real cause—that is, if they communicate the power which performs vital functions and produces vital vigor—there will be an "invariable connection" between the drug and the function. There will be no function with the drug; and there will be an increase or decrease of function corresponding to any increase or decrease of the drug. The absurdity of such a claim is evident; it rests only on superstition sustained by indifference.. ." (*Vital Science*, p. 263.)

It is the body that acts, and not the drug, serum, or body waste. It is the danger inherent in the poisonous nature of these things that prompts the body to act. The action is in self-defense, and is produced by a calling out of the body's reserve forces; just as the danger of the enemy prompted the man to act in self-defense, and struggle until his strength was exhausted. The effects of the abnormal action are beating heart, throbbing brain, rapid respiration, profuse perspiration, vomiting, diarrhoea, skin eruptions, fever, etc. The nature and locality of the symptoms is what determines the name the physicians give them, and that is incidental and immaterial. The more poisonous any substance is, the more dangerous it is, and the quicker and harder the body acts—sending a large dose of salts or castor oil through the alimentary canal with a rush. Such treatment, instead of its being curative, is destructive; for it is a terrible shock to the nervous system, and may be continued until the body will utterly collapse from the exhaustion induced by its own violent efforts of self-protection.

From what has been said and shown, we observe how clear it is that the first and only step to be taken in the prevention and "cure" of any "disease," is to obey the Law. But the thought that obeying the Law of Life rebounds to one's greatest good now and forever, seems never to have entered into man's philosophy. The Law of Life is the Law of the Universe; the Law of the Universe is the Law of God. The road to an understanding of God and His work, is from the seed to the plant, and from the plant to the seed again.

We repeat: Here is the profound principle from which Great Nature operates. Medical science (?) has made many "discoveries," but here is one that has been overlooked, in spite of all the brilliant workers, their super-education, their vast expenditures of money, their endless research work, experiments, sacrifice of life, and so on. At the Center is Simplicity and Unity of cause (the Life Principle), while at the Surface is Infinite Variety of Appearance of sickness, exhibited in the various and mystifying symptom complexes of disease, termed mumps, measles, catarrh, eczema, pneumonia, typhoid, smallpox, cancer, and so on, which infinite Variety of Appearance "scientists" have been studying, naming, and treating for thirty centuries, and to which they have attached the highest importance, while the Simplicity and Unity of Cause at the Center remains neglected, unknown, and obscure.

Medical science (?) has never studied nor investigated anything pertaining to "disease," except the Infinite Variety of Appearance at the surface, which they have done to the total exclusion of all else. These they study, name, and treat, while the Simplicity and Unity of Cause at the Center is entirely ignored and utterly disregarded. For thirty centuries they have thought entirely from the eye (appearance), and this has blinded their understanding and closed up their will; and from a freedom that is in accord with its reason, the will does only that which has been confirmed in the understanding. The understanding is blinded not only by ignorance, but equally by false doctrine. For as Truths open the understanding, so Falsities close it up.

It follows from what has been said and shown, that sickness comes from within, not without. Sickness indicates the effect of the Life Principle within, actively engaged in trying to save the body from destruction. The kind of sickness—the surface symptoms—while resulting from the Unity of Cause at the Center, may be and is as variable at the surface, as to medical diagnosis, as are the winds of the earth, or the products of the soil. We may diagnose these symptoms—Variety of Appearance at the Surface—as mumps, measles, catarrh, consumption, cancer, smallpox, etc., as we similarly name the various products of the soil as wheat, corn, oats, many kinds of grasses, weeds, trees, etc.; but regardless of the arbitrary names of the symptoms at the surface, they all come from and center in one cause!

When we know the principles from which Nature operates, and realize that ALL illness comes from Unity of Cause at the Center (poisoned blood), regardless of the medical names of the infinite Variety of Appearance at the Surface, we then understand how fruitless it is to name these symptoms (diagnosis), and how useless it is to treat and suppress these symptoms (therapeutics). Useless did we say? Destructive is a far better and more fitting term.

The healer who knows the principles from which Nature operates, puts no dependence in such changeable and unreliable signs as symptoms, and cares less for their medical names. He directs his attention not to these, since they have to do only with effects, and not with the Unity of Cause at the Center. Cause is one thing and effect is another. The difference between the two is similar to the difference between prior and subsquent, or between that which forms and that which is formed. Effects may be studied to eternity, but such process will not reveal the cause. That is why all medical practice books state that—

"the cause of disease is unknown;"

and why Dr. Osler, England's greatest physician, declared—

"of (the cause of) disease we know nothing at all."

God is cause and man is effect. We may study man (effect) to eternity, and yet know nothing regarding God (cause). Every effect is visible, while every cause is invisible, and can be discovered, not by studying effects, but—

Only by keeping the understanding for a long time in spiritual light.

When we study effects, we think from the eye; in the study of cause we must necessarily think from the understanding, since causes are invisible. But medical men study effects, and think from the eye, and of such people Swedenborg observes—

They think from the eye, and are not able to think from the understanding. Thought from the eye closes the understanding, but thought from understanding opens the eyes.

Accordingly, the healer who thinks from the understanding (cause at the center), and not from the eye (appearance at the surface), understands the principles from which Nature operates and directs his efforts to the Unity of Cause at the Center (blood), and not to the Variety of Appearance at the Surface (symptoms). When the Unity of Cause at the Center (blood), grown normal because of right living, and never because of any treatment, medical or otherwise, the Infinite Variety of Appearance at the Surface will wither and die, as the plants in a field after their roots have been cut asunder. These plants in a field, after their roots have been severed, wither and die regardless of their names. The surface symptoms of illness may be diagnosed as mumps, measles, catarrh, cancer, smallpox, and so on, but they cannot live and thrive when the blood has been clarified and purified. They must wither, die, and disappear.

The whole matter may be properly summarized as follows:

1—Life is the creative force functioning in the body. In health it functions smoothly and silently. When its function is obstructed, it struggles to save the body by conquering the obstructing object or condition. This struggle is termed disease and named according to location of symptoms. There is no such thing as disease per se.

2—The continuous and harmonious existence of the body depends upon strict compliance with Law of Life written in every particle of its structure.

3—The body is created complete and perfect, wanting in nothing, and incapable of receiving anything from human hands. It is self-operating, self-regulating, self-repairing, self-preserving, and self-curing.

4—All the healing power in the Universe is within the body.

5—No power, force, substance, or thing is able to save the body or serve the healing power within, further than to remove the obstruction responsible for its disturbed equilibrium.

6—The life of the flesh is in the blood. The life of all flesh is the blood thereof (Lev. 17:11,14).

7—Insofar as the blood remains active and normal, and to that degree only, will and must all organs, tissues, and cells remain healthy and normal.

The life of all flesh is the blood thereof, and as the condition of the blood is, so must the flesh be. For as the continuous existence of the body is dependent wholly upon the blood, it must follow that good health or poor health depends upon and springs from the blood. So the vital stream that turns the wheels of life is not only the health-producing and life-sustaining power, but also the disease-producing and life-destroying power. It could not be otherwise without reversing law and order. Therefore, the healer who knows the principles from which Nature operates, takes the following position:

1—The continuous existence of the body depends upon the blood.

2—A normal flow of normal blood brings health.

3—Retarded circulation and foul, impure blood brings disease.

4—Purification of the blood and acceleration of the circulation is scientific treatment. There can be no other.

5—The means to accomplish this are supplied by the body alone. The body makes blood and purifies it. Nothing else can do this work.

6—The supply determines the method of procedure.

7—The procedure must be natural; and, being natural, results are and must be favorable and permanent.

Everything in the Universe is governed by Law. If we know the law and apply it, there invariably follows results so certain as to be amazing because of their positiveness. We can prevision and predict, with perfect accuracy, the results of certain actions and conditions. This is the Law of Cause and Effect. Man has applied this Law with startling success to many things, but seems never to have considered applying it to his own body. Does man, in his pride and vanity, believe that he is so far apart from Nature that Nature's laws apply not to him? Is he too proud to acknowledge obedience to his Master? The proper application of

God's Law is merely obedience to His command; and by strictly obeying the Law, man eliminates all uncertainty as to disease, just as he, in the same way eliminates all uncertainty as to all other things; and Health then flows as silently, freely, and naturally, as the tide rises and falls. Why not? They are all governed by the same Law!

. . . "Fortunately, there exists a healing art which has been found very efficient as a means of removing disease, and restoring the body to a condition of health. It is distinguished from medical science, chiropractic, osteopathy and all other schools, sects and systems of healing, both in theory and in practice. It is concerned with removing the cause of disease, whereas others are content to treat the end-points of disease. In this sense it belongs in a class by itself. It is diametrically opposed to all other healing arts.

"This unusual science of healing is known as the Hygienic System. It was developed a little more than a century ago in the United States by Isaac Jennings, M. D., Russel Thacher Trall, M. D., and Sylvester Graham. These three men presented their new theories of healtl. and disease in a wide array of publications. These include: *Medical Reform, Philosophy of Human Life* and *Tree of Life, or Human Degeneracy, Its Nature and Remedy, as Based on the Elevating Principles of Orthopathy, by Dr. Jennings; The Hygienic System, Hydropathic Encyclopedia, The Hygienic Handbook, Sexual Physicology, Popular Physiology, Hydropathy for the People, Mother's Hygienic Handbook, Scientific Basis of Vegetarianism, Digestion and Dyspepsia, Diseases of the Throat and Lungs, The Alcoholic Controversy, Hydropathic Cook-Book, Illustrated Family Gymnasium* and others by Dr. Trall; and *Health from Diet and Exercise, Nature's Own Book* and *Lectures on the Science of Human Life* by *Sylvester Graham.* These publications were the foundation of early hygienic practice. They also provided a basis for the future development of the Hygienic System.

"After the death of Jennings, Trall and Graham, others took up the cause of the Hygienic System. They established a number of sanatoriums throughout America where they carried on the work of applying the hygienic methods in the treatment of disease. The knowledge gained from this experience formed the basis of a new array of publications which were released intermittently up to the present day. Included among these are: *How to Treat the Sick Without Drugs, Hygienic Medication or Science Versus Speculation and Nature's Method of Curing the Sick by James C. Jackson, M. D.; The Nutritive Cure, Hygienic Hydropathy, Exact Science of Health, Life's Greatest Law, Philosophy of Health Reform, A Defense of Hygienic Treatment, How Sick People Are Cured, and Drug Medicines as Causes of Disease by Robert Walter, M. D.; The Bible of Nature, Body and Mind, Physical Education and Fasting, Hydrotherapy and Exercise by Felix L. Oswald; Paralysis and Other Affections of the Nerves, and An Exposition of the Swedish Movement Cure by George H. Taylor; Life and Health or the Laws and Means of Physical Culture by William A. Alcott, M. D.; Drugless Medicine by Susanna W. Dodds, M. D.; The Natural Cure by Charles E. Page; How Nature Cures*

and Natural Cure of Consumption by Emmet Densmore; The No-Break-
fast Plan and Fasting Cure and The True Science of Living by Edward
Hooker Dewey, M. D.; The Genesis and Control of Disease by George S.
Weger, M. D.; Criticisms of the Practice of Medicine, Impaired Health,
and Toxemia Explained by John H. Tilden, M. D.; and The Hygienic
System (seven volumes) by Herbert M. Shelton. These works, though
only a fraction of those which have been published, have exerted a great
influence in developing the Hygienic System to its present position. Most
of them are now out of print; of the authors, only Herbert M. Shelton
is still living.

"Though the Hygienic System originated over a century ago, it has
taken until now for it to develop into its position as a truly scientific
healing art. In its modern phase it is the product of the accumulated
knowledge acquired by hygienists throughout the last century. It was
never discovered as such, but simply developed year by year through
continued experience and observation. The Hygienic System of the
nineteenth century was obviously not as efficient as that of today. It
had the same basic premises, but its practical application had yet to be
perfected. In fact, it can still be improved. However, we have gone
most of the way. Splendid health, both in youth and old age, is now
possible. The Hygienic System has scored a major victory.

"The Hygienic System opens up the possibility of an entirely new
phase of life for the human race. In consideration of what already has
been discovered, it has become necessary to entirely reconsider and
revaluate all past conceptions relating to prevention of disease, removal
of disease, preservation of youth, and the length of life. We are no longer
justified in dividing disease into so-called curable and incurable types.
Nor are we justified in speaking of the inevitability of senility and a
human life span which is much shorter, in accordance with the time
required to reach maturity, than is the general rule in the animal kingdom. The removal of most manifestations of existing disease, the prevention of at least 95 per cent of all disease, a life span of 100 to 150
years, the preservation of youthful vitality, and the occurrence of pain-
less death, probably during sleep, in a very advanced life—these are the
probable results of the Hygienic System when applied to the human
species to the fullest extent over the required period of time. The full
and complete employment of the Hygienic System in tens of thousands
of cases, as well as extensive observations and studies in the field of
physiology, biology, chemistry, anthropology, anthropogenesis, paleon-
tology, and zoology, provide a sound, scientific basis for these statements.

"Since the time of Jennings, Trall and Graham, the Hygienic System
has been the victim of many attacks. Its exponents have always been
called faddists and quacks. Many of them have served prison sentences
and have been heavily fined for employing hygienic methods in the
treatment of disease. Others have been mobbed while making lectures.
The uprisings were usually inspired by commercial enterprises which
saw, in the Hygienic System, a danger to their vested interests.

"Medical science has been particularly active in fighting this science
of healing. It has always referred to hygienists as quacks, and has fre-

quently prevented them from practicing. However, it has never made any official investigations to determine the results of hygienic practice. Medical science saw in the Hygienic System, as did other commercial enterprises, a danger to its financial interests. This has no doubt been partly responsible for its antagonistic attitude. Had hygienic practice been commercially profitable, it might have been absorbed into medical practice.

"There are no hygienic practitioners who have been trained as such. The only hygienists are medical or drugless physicians who have dropped the practices of their profession and taken up those of the Hygienic System. Dr. Trall established the only college which trained students to be Hygienists and it lasted only a short time. It did not establish the Hygienic System as a profession, but rather conferred the degree M. D., upon graduation. As a legalized profession the Hygienic System has never had any real existence. The hygienist has always had to practice under the guise of medical science, chiropractic, or some other healing art.

"This state of affairs is undesirable because it limits the number of hygienists to a very small figure. However, it does not prevent the majority of people from making a practical application of the Hygienic System. This healing art differs from all others in the sense that its employment usually does not require professional supervision. Its simplicity and safety make it an effective tool in the hands of the layman. A professional status would be valuable chiefly for research and educational purposes. Once the knowledge of the Hygienic System became widespread it would (with rare exceptions) be self applied. The present need for a larger number of professional hygienists would then disappear. The profession would remain, but only on a very small scale."
—*The Fountain of Youth*, by Arnold DeVries by special permission of the author).

EXTRACTS FROM LETTERS
BY EMINENT HEALTH REFORMERS
Hereward Carrington, Ph.D.

During my early days, when writing my books on fasting and diet, I carried on a fairly voluminous correspondence with many of the exponents of hygiene then active, including Dr. Dewey, Dr. Rabagliati, Dr. Oswald, and others. Thinking that such extracts from their letters might be of interest, they are reproduced herewith, hoping that they may be considered of historical value. The originals are in my possession, and the quotations may be verified by any serious student of the subject.

LETTERS
FROM DR. EDWARD HOOKER DEWEY

Jan. 3, 1903

My Dear Mr. Carrington:
    Very glad to hear from you, and shall be glad to get any new points evolved by your experience. I want to advise you to procure Horace Fletcher's 'New Glutton or Epicure.' It is the best book for all to read, who are still able to eat, that has ever been penned by mortal man!
                    Very truly,   E. H. DEWEY

Feb. 21, 1903

    I am very, very pleased to hear from you — and to assure you that I consider the case of Mr. Davis the most remarkable case I know of on record as a revelation of Nature's power over disease. I have long held that a fast, if long enough, would cure such diseases. The physiology of it is this: Through the fast the clot that was, originally, had changed into an organized mass that pressed upon the nerve-roots; hence the paralysis: this mass became softer, so as to be absorbed as brain-food. In this way cancers and other diseased structures are eaten up as brain food. . . . I hope to know you better. . . .

March 26, 1903

    Only God could break a fast where there is a sick stomach and there is no time to let Nature perform the task. Taking food into such a stomach is death-dealing. There is nothing to do but to make the body and mind as comfortable as possible, and Nature will cure, if the seal of death is not set.
    In the case you referred to, of death, the vomiting was stopped not by the food taken, but by an event or condition in the history of this disease. Death was inevitable *shortly*, and if only broth or some liquid food had been taken, only to be vomited up, the patient would have suffered more and died sooner; but the friends would have been better satisfied! Do you see the point?

I am very pleased to hear from you again. . . . As to the doctors: They, as a class, have average honesty; they treat disease to the best of their knowledge and ability. There is no treatment in any book that recognizes the brain as a self-feeding organ, in time of sickness or starvation, as the source of the strength of the body—and that is only kept-up by rest and sleep. No book that recognizes digestion and assimilation as a tax upon the brain. Hence the utter confusion over this vast matter of the nutrition of the body, and the source and maintenance of the strength. Think of Mark Hanna being awakened every two hours, during the night before his death, to be fed, to "keep up his strength!"

Now as to your fasting theories: I must inform you that I cannot now recall that I ever put any patient on a fast in a physiological sense. I have always been dealing with cases of abolished hunger from mental or physical diseases. Fasts are instituted by Nature. They begin with the loss of appetite and end with hunger; and all the suffering involved is due to disease, and not in the least to lack of the ordinary daily food.

This must be held as exactly true in all acute diseases. There is a great deal of habit-want in all eating, with stimulation the first impression; hence the vital powers are thrown into some confusion when the food-supply is cut off, somewhat as when habitual stimulants are abolished. In a strict physiological sense, fasting is a resting process for the vital powers, to the extent of stopping for the time the use of the hardest machine to run—the stomach. Normal digestion causes a degree of mental torpor; this becomes habitual in all cases of indigestion. Once the stomach and bowels become empty, as during a fast, Nature becomes more keenly alive to her wrongs, and is in a condition more clearly to express them. Hence the suffering for a time when the habits are given up.

But the brain feeds itself and regains power, as it cannot if any is diverted to the stomach. Voluntary fasting involves more or less depressing apprehension. This is so inevitable that I do not advise any to go on protracted fasts when I cannot have their personal care. . . .

Now let me repeat: The brain can keep itself fully nourished without a morsel of food until the body is reduced to a skeleton—without one abnormal mental symptom, when no disease is involved. . . . Fasting then is only a resting of the brain from the use of the hardest machine in the entire body to run. More than twenty-six years in the rooms of the sick have proved this to my complete satisfaction.

I should be pleased if you would let me know of any of your articles that are appearing. The last one of my own was in "Physical Culture," of December, in response to one by a Dr. Lawson, on "The Errors in the Fasting Cure," in the November number.

With kindest wishes . . . .

March 25, 1904

From some new light that has been coming to me, I am becoming more and more convinced that it requires so little food to maintain normal weight that we can get it out of almost any of the ordinary foods. The great question is one of such thorough mastication as to reduce the labor of both brain and stomach to their lowest terms.

It may be taken for granted, that any bill of fare that is deficient in nourishment, so that the weight declines unduly, will be attended by an increasing demand for food, and it will be very likely to be of the more nourishing kinds. I think this is the experience in cases of famine.

My objection to meat as an article of diet is that it contains very little nourishment, and that what there is, is hard to convert into flesh and blood. The fiber is practically indigestible. It cannot be reduced to liquid by mastication. It is probably the most expensive of all the more common foods. . . .

The greatest of all troubles that come from our daily food is from 'bolting' and excess above the need. This more than the quality of it. I object to your method (fruitarianism) because it is not practical. The great mass of the world's people have no time, taste or even ability to theorize along dietetic lines. And then most of them subsist upon foods that are the most available along their geographical lines. I have felt from the first that I did the best I could for the people, that is, the most that would be practical for me, when I induced them to give up their morning meals. I early found out that the sharp contrast between the forenoon clearness, cheer and energy, and after-dinner sluggishness, was always a matter of discipline, tending to lessen gluttony. . . . I have not the slightest doubt of your ability to keep your body perfectly nourished on fruit and nut foods. . . .

I am so taken-up just now by the building of an addition to my house, and by the unusual addition to my correspondence, that I am not able to write as I would to you. I shall be pleased to have you point out any further errors you find in any of my books, articles or letters. . . . I have only changed along dietetic lines in that I now realize, as not formerly, that less food is required to meet the demands of waste than I had believed, and that the average amount can be greatly reduced by thorough mastication. . . .

June 15, 1904

From Mrs. Dewey

That Dr. Dewey seemingly neglected the correspondence with you, had a very grevious cause. My poor husband had a stroke of apoplexy on the 28th of March, which paralyzed his right side and bereft him of speech for some time. What the cause of his stroke was who can say? The Doctor had never been sick, and had most probably gone beyond his strength. For months he has been under an unusual mental strain. In February we had a runaway with the cutter, in which I was considerably hurt. The doctor did not complain, but I noticed for days after that, nervous contractions in his legs. Several professional trips followed that robbed him of his sleep for almost a week.

It is the most pitiful sight: this man whom everybody knew as ever alert, active, from the very early morning (he hardly ever rose later than

4 o'clock), full of life—now helpless, broken down, emaciated. He improved seemingly rapidly in the beginning, but about two weeks ago he began to fail. We can hardly look forward to a recovery, though he may live yet for some time; he is now in a drowsy condition most of the time. . . .

August 11, 1904

From A. J. Dewey

Mrs. Dewey has asked me to write you, as at present she is incapacitated. After consultation we decided to take both the doctor and Mrs. Dewey to the hospital here for several weeks: she to rest-up, and he for the care he would otherwise miss at home. All Mrs. Dewey needs is complete rest for a while, and this she will get. The doctor is making no particular progress lately. He cannot walk, although he sits up in a wheel chair every day and reads considerably. His nights are very restless. . . . I do not know if there is anything of importance to tell, but will gladly answer your kindly inquiries at any time. . . .

August 22, 1904

From Mrs. Dewey

My dear patient has been improving lately, both physically and mentally. The chief cause of my worry for him, this last week, has been the bloating of his face. The kidneys do not work right. Since Saturday I have used applications of cold water. . . . He is very much stronger, is in his chair almost all day long, eats with us at the table, using his right hand. . . . In his mind he is also much better; the chief weakness is in his short memory; he often has forgotten ten minutes after his meal that he has eaten. Like all apoplectic people, he has a good appetite—too good an appetite—but I have no difficulty in restricting it. I have simply to convince him that his memory plays him a trick, and that his is a sham appetite. . . .

I cannot remember whether I have given you any details of his sickness, but at the risk of repeating myself, I will say that, after his stroke, he fasted for 4 or 5 weeks; then lived a long time on broth. After his second stroke he had again several days of fasting and of very little eating. Toast and a soft egg and a dish of broth was all he ate during the day; only recently has he craved a variety of food, being thoroughly tired of broth. His nights are better, too, though he does not sleep an hour during the whole night. He takes now an interest in the letters that come, and he reads the papers every day. . . . I wish we had a better climate here. . . . He fasted for *weeks* after his stroke, much to the distress of the physician who attended him — fasted till hunger and a clean tongue came. I will write you shortly. . . .

Dec. 16, 1904

The pitiful thing has happened. My poor doctor has had a third stroke. . . . for three and a half hours he had the most awful convulsions; then he fell into a state of coma, lasting 36 hours; he is now very low; the left side is now paralyzed; hope seems impossible.

Accept the assurance of my full appreciation of the sincere sympathy you expressed in your letter. When the fatal news had to be sent out, I added your name to the list — so you have been informed about the end of our beloved one. But you may wish more particulars, and I am very glad to speak about the doctor to anyone who has as sincere an interest in the doctor and his work as I know you have.

You cannot understand how the doctor failed to recover; it seems, indeed, incredible, when his constitution, during all his sickness, seemed so wonderful as to baffle all the physicians, who frankly admitted that such marvelous vitality could only be due to his strict habits of life.

After his third stroke his attending physician expected the end every night, and so did all the other physicians who came in to see him; after a few days they did not venture an opinion any more.

I who have watched him so closely for many months have come to the conclusion that his peculiar nervous condition, that prevented his sleep and his cure, was caused chiefly by his worry about himself. He understood his own case only too well; he watched every symptom of it, although he hardly ever spoke of it. He who was used to never-ceasing activity could not reconcile himself to being tied to the chair—to being unable to use his beloved pen. Then he realized and worried over his finances—to be cut off from all income; he worried over the future, etc., though we all tried our best to make him feel at rest about such matters. He had never been sick (except when, as a young man, he suffered from indigestion); hence he had no training in enduring a long illness and awaiting his recovery with patience. This, I think, is quite an important factor.

The end came without any struggle, and the face, in the calmness of death, looked serene and noble and beautiful. I am glad to remember this face so fully at rest, with the dignity of victory.

Thanking you once more for your letter. . . .

This is in reply to your friendly letter, for which I am very grateful to you. . . . I certainly agree with you in your view as to the influence of mental conditions on the health of the body. . . . He was too great a man to worry about everything; he was, for example, singularly unconcerned about the criticisms and ridicule he received in return for his books and doctrines. . . . Nevertheless he had many, many cares and troubles, and if he did not allow himself to worry and fret over them, they were ever there, to weigh down on him. And a never-ending activity—overwork constantly; it was work that he loved, but which he could never consider a pastime, because he was dependent upon the fruits of it for his daily bread.

This is the first news I have had of your writing a book on fasting; I shall be exceedingly interested in it. I send you with this mail a remarkable record of a fast. Mr. Patterson has kindly consented to allow me to use it as I see fit. I have no doubt that it will be very interesting to you. . . .

I am very sorry not to have seen you again when in New York. Business prevented. I expect to leave on Monday. Thanking you again for your interest.....

Kathe N. Dewey

FROM DR. HENRY S. TANNER
(THE DR. TANNER!)

Feb. 11, 1908

I received your letter yesterday. Just now I am very busy getting material together for a book I am publishing soon. Then I will gladly avail myself of the opportunity to aid you in your good work of spreading the glad tidings of the therapeutic value of fasting. I esteem it among the very best of means of helping sick and discouraged humanity to regain its health, physically and mentally. I have found it such, and cheerfully recommend it to all in like need.

FROM CHARLES C. HASKELL

June 7, 1905

Through Mr. J. Austin Shaw, who has been fasting for 45 days, I have learned of your interest in the subject, and that you are preparing a work upon fasting, that will doubtless be interesting and profitable to all humanity. I should be glad to know more about it. I am deeply and vitally interested in the redemption of humanity from diseases, and any contribution that is made to the stock of knowledge that we already have would be deeply interesting to me. . . .

June 14, 1905

I was much pleased to receive your letter, telling me so fully concerning the book you are preparing. I know it will be a valuable contribution to health literature, and helpful in showing many the way to health and life. Some of the books you mention I have; others I have not. . . . If I can be of service to you in any way, in the matter of helping you to get such facts as you desire for publication, I am at your service. I hope I may hear again from you. . . .

FROM J. AUSTIN SHAW

June 5, 1905

I have your letter. . . . Kindly note the references to my fast in last Friday's "Herald"; they are the most nearly correct. You are at liberty to utilize the information therein given. I expect to write an account of it for one of the Sunday papers, and am writing a book, giving my daily experiences. In this I cover the points you mention. Later, I hope to lecture on the subject, and perhaps fast while doing so. . . .

June 15, 1905

I found your letter on my return from Norwich, where I visited Mr. Haskell. I am glad you wrote him. . . . Thanks for your advice. I think you are right about the inadvisability of fasting during a lecture course; also about not taking another fast immediately. I have only gained 2 pounds since the fast ended. In other words, adding to it— just enough to supply the daily waste. . . .

(Brief letters from Dr. Emmet Densmore, Horace Fletcher, Eustace Miles, and others—hardly worth quoting, however).

FROM DR. FELIX OSWALD

Oct. 21, 1903

Your friendly letter received—almost the first of its kind from your great city, though scores of sympathetic communications reach me from rural districts, every month. Verily health, like freedom, is a nymph of the mountains and ocean-cliffs. . . . I enclose a partial list of my literary sins. I am getting out an edition of my hygienic writings, in uniform binding, and if you are interested, shall be pleased to forward you a set with my compliments. . . .

Sept. 3, 1904

A day after the receipt of your last letter I had a chat with a veteran librarian who tried in vain to recollect any monograph on the subject of Fasting, and then dived into his stack of Catalogs, but still shook his head. "Nothing extant on that exclusive subject in English." So you may be right, and have a certainly not-understood theme all to your-self—as a specialized study, I mean. . . .

FROM DR. SUSANNA W. DODDS

June 21, 1904

. . . . I am glad you are interested in hygiene. I am myself a Trall graduate, and I know that a knowledge of his teachings has been the means of saving not only my own life (I am in my seventy-fourth year) but that of many of my friends. There is nothing wrong with the *principles* which Trall taught. . . .

I did not know that Louis Kuhne was dead. When did that happen? Nor did I know that Dr. Reinhold had passed away, until I saw a notice of the "late" Dr. Reinhold. Can you give me any particulars in his case?

As to Dr. Dewey, I have never read his books thoroughly. I have heard that he drank coffee, ate meat, white bread, etc., and if he in-dulged in hearty suppers, I see no reason why he should not fall a victim to apoplexy. I believe he discarded fruits, especially the acid varieties, almost entirely. He was certainly not a hygienist. . . .

I think that, in trying to profit by the instructions of our health reformers, it is well to avoid copying their faults and mistakes; none of these men are perfect. . . . I used to ask Trall why he sat up late at night when he advised others to do differently. He replied that his time was so occupied through the day, and he was interrupted in so many ways, that night was the only time that things were quiet and he could do his writings. He ought to have lived twenty or thirty years longer than he did.

We have been in practice for nearly thirty-five years, and we do not give drug medicines to our patients. We believe in Trall's teachings, that drug poisons kill, not cure. . . .

July 23, 1904

. . . Did I, in my letter, speak of "catching" cold? If so, the language was very unphysiological. What is usually termed a cold is but the result of broken law. It is NOT effort. As Trall used to teach us, disease (remedial effort) unless *directed* intelligently, may lead to a fatal termination. It is the work of the true physician (the hygienist) not to suppress remedial effort, as the drug-doctors are doing with their medicines, but to control and direct it. His object should be so to balance vital action in every part of the living organism that life will not be endangered . . .

I thoroughly approve of the no-breakfast plan for those who eat hearty suppers. For myself, I greatly prefer the two meal system, the last one being taken not later than 3 or 4 p.m.; and *both* meals to be earned before they are eaten.

Very few there are who can grasp these hygienic principles in their entirety. Trall was a believer in fasting, within limits, of course . . .

July 24, 1905

I see that you are very sympathetic with Trall and his teachings. I regard him as the leading spirit in the nineteenth century. No other writer grasped the subject, the true healing art, as he did.

Yes, I too am disgusted when I hear people say that 'only in the gravest cases' would they give medicine—which merely proves that they don't know the alphabet, either as to what disease is, or how to cure the sick. They simply do not know what they are talking about . . .

FROM DR. A. RABAGLIATI

Oct. 7, 1904

I am very much interested in your letter,—about disease being a condition of the body and not an entity. We doctors deal with conditions of body, and as we find much difficulty, or even impossibility in defining health, so we find equal difficulty in defining disease, which is any and every departure from health . . . On the whole you are correct; but who has been more insistent than I, in showing that it is not, e.g., microorganisms which are important, as growing in the body, but rather the state of the body which harbors and makes them grow? And therefore, as I say, I do not admit that tuberculosis is caused by the growth in the body of the tub. bacilli, but I contend that tuberculosis is the state of the body which makes the bacillus grow and thrive in it. A most essential difference this, which most seem incapable of understanding.

I have often said that I should be ashamed to have influenza, and that, if I had influenza with pneumonia, I should be disgraced. Because in that case I know I should have been over-fed, and that, in the latter case, I had been grossly over-fed. So I say about taking colds; in fact I am fast getting to that state of mind, as regards cancer, or rather, as I should prefer to say, becoming cancerous, or getting into the cancerous state. I am sure that we 'eat cancer' . . .

I am greatly interested in what you say about the quantity of food required by the body, and how your conclusions agree with mine. I think Prof. Chittenden's experiments have settled that. We eat twice or thrice what we require. But I do not think you will prove your theory of energy—or at least find it accepted. You will have your task cut out, and I don't envy you!

It's a case of Carrington *contra mundam!*

Nov. 6, 1904

. . . Now I come to the main topic of this letter. The suggestion that food has no relation to energy-production (directly) in the human body is of the very highest and deepest interest. The suggestion does not, and need not in the least, contravene the law of the conservation of energy. The question may be put in this form: Is not the human body much more analogous in its working to an electric motor than it is to a steam engine? The steam engine undoubtedly transforms the potential energy of the coal or fuel into kinetic energy, in the form of work done, put the energy it receives into work. If the coal remade and re-formed the mechanism of the engine, instead of wearing and burning it up, it would perform in the engine the function that food performs in the body . . . Well, that seems to me a very fine suggestion! It has every appearance of being correct on this view, the chief function of the 'engineer' in the body is to keep the machinery in good order, — all the points clean and bright, so to speak, — in order that the energy everywhere about us in illimitable quantity may enter in, according to the capacity of each of feeding—which is required, not to change food into work, but to change us; and the chief way to keep the machine in good order is by proper food into body, and to maintain the body so as to make it a good transmitter or transformer of energy. Oh, it is a fine theory!

You might perhaps put your theory otherwise. Food bears to mentality the same relation that oxygen bears to flame. It supports flame, but does not itself burn; and the body transmits and transforms energy, but is not itself the source of it,—through metabolism. What a wonderful idea; And how much more important than ever—that the body should be properly fed, and not choked so by over-feeding or improper feeding, that its energy cannot get in, in order to be transmitted and transformed . . .

Dec. 18, 1904

Your two letters have interested me greatly. I am a little sorry for having mentioned your idea, since you wished to be the first to announce it. But so far as I am concerned I have humbly given you priority in announcement, and no one shall ever deprive you of the honor with my good will. I would give anything to have been the originator of such an idea, or to have been deemed worthy by the all-inspiring spirit to have such an idea entrusted or suggested to me—an idea so far-reaching, so beautiful, so revolutionary, so unlikely to be suggested to anyone in the present gross, material condition of science, which to my mind has so strangely deprived itself of philosophy . . . But when I did have such an idea presented me, how could I hold my peace about it? To me the mere statement of it carries with it its own proof, or the conviction of its truth; but I know too well that science will demand what it calls proof, and of course we must be prepared with proof of the sort demanded . . . I sent one copy of my paper to a medical journal, but I need hardly say they would not print it! It is a most revolutionary idea; I wonder if you realize how revolutionary it is? Thanks for all the books and papers . . .

. . . As to the internal and external work of the body: I think you are right. They are phases of the same thing. The motions of the heart and vessels, like the motion of the muscles, are not dependent upon the food at all, in the way usually believed. The sole function of food is to repair the machine *through* which, and not *by* which, the work is done. Obviously, if this be so, the quantity of food required, is far less than we doctors have been in the habit of telling the public,—we having been indoctrinated by the physiologists. Chittenden's book puts this practical conclusion most forcibly,—although throughout his book, he never seems to have a glimmer, even faint, of this grand, underlying idea you have given me, and which seems to have fascinated and carried me away.

Jan. 7, 1906

I am content to wait till your book is ready, though I hope it will not be too long, as I think this idea should go out to the world . . . Don't fast too much. There is reason in all things. Sixteen hours' work a day means waste,—even if the energy does not come from food,—and this needs replacement. For my sake don't kill yourself! I think you have the most valuable idea in your mind that, in this department, the world has ever heard of, and I should grieve sorely if it had to be referred to as a valuable suggestion or contribution to science by "a late young and talented author!" Old fellows like me can stand much more than young ones. I have always been a delicate man, but I can stand almost anything in the way of fatigue . . .

Patients gain weight in fasting (in one way) by absorbing water, and using-up exudation in connective tissue, replacing this by larger quantities of water. Coincidentally, such patients get much less stiff and tender,—proving, I think, the absorption of the exudation which causes the tenderness . . . Thanks again for your very interesting letter.

March 25, 1906

I have read over two or three times all your brilliant papers, and I must congratulate you very much. You have given me at least two new ideas of the most supreme importance: First, that the combustion of food is probably not the source of the mechanical energy of the body, and Second, that neither is it probably the source of the heat of the body. The latter is the more marvelous. I don't suppose that science will

— 91 —

humbly cave-in and admit that she is wrong, but if true, these things will one day be proved . . . I think you have worked-out the question of sub-normal temperature admirably, and I think you are right in this. . .

August 15, 1907

. . . You say you are at work on your book again. You must get it out! This theory is the most important ever launched in physiology, in fact, it at once shows that all the stuff about "calories" is pretentious nonsense. What could be more important than this? You have helped to open my eyes with a vengeance, and I imagine I am getting them wider opened even than yours. I am working on a new theory of energy; we'll see!

Nov. 2, 1907

Thanks for your long letter and also the proofs of the book, which have now arrived. I am going through them carefully and will begin my Introduction soon. Only you must give me a little time. This is the most serious controversy ever raised in physiology, for it involves nothing less than a new theory of energy. Let me congratulate you on the completeness and feeling of discrimination of your book. It ought to revolutionize thinking and practice . . . And you have not only raised the question, but solved it!

December 10, 1907

. . . So far as I can make out, this energy of the body must be akin to the Eastern "prana." One of its forms is vital energy; but there seems to be a prana of substance, as well as of the body; and I think it is an advantage to name these different forms of energy separately,—not forgetting for a moment that they are different forms of the same power. Prana might perhaps be called Spirit, when it takes the form of bio-dynamic energy. . . . But the soul or Ego? I hardly like to write it, but I think perhaps this might be a spark of God himself. One is awed, overpowered, by such a suggestion. Truly the inquiry is infinite and endless. . . . . .

July 26, 1908

. . . This controversy of ours on the theory of energy will not be settled for many years, doubtless; but we have done our part. And the same Power which produces us will continue to carry-on its own purpose through others, who will arise in the future. So, be of good cheer!

June 5, 1912

Many thanks for your book "The Natural Food of Man," which I have read with great interest. . . Regarding the question of the rate of circulation of blood in the brain; I am sure it is a fact that this moves coincidentally with the respiriation and not coincidentally with the heart-beat. For proofs of this see R. L. Tafel: "The Brain Considered Automatically, Physiologically and Philosophically," London, 1887. Vol. 1, pp. 645-700, contains his most elaborate and learned Note on this subject. All the authorities of any importance are cited. I have read and re-read it, and am convinced that he had proved that the brain-circulation is not coincidental with the blood-circulation, but the respiration. . . . This is most significant, if true.

I so enjoyed your visit when you came to England, and hope we may meet again some day. . . . .

A. Rabagliati

EXTRACTS FROM A LETTER OF MINE
TO DR. RABAGLIATI

May 8, 1905

Dear Dr. Rabagliati:

Your kind post-card received, and I quite appreciate the fact that your correspondence must be extensive and heavy, and must ask you not to consider writing to me until you have some leisure on your hands. . . . .

I do not know if you are especially interested in Psychical Research topics, but they are, after all, the borderland-phenomena, and the connecting link between science and philosophy. I have just finished an article on the origin and nature of consciousness, which I will send you as soon as out. It may interest you, perhaps.

Coming now to the more prosaic subject of diet, Chittenden's book is of course valuable, but I doubt if it will be a popular book! I am of course much pleased by your remarks about the energy of the body in relation to food. . . . After all, what is the difference between internal and external work? Do they not both depend upon the expenditure of energy? Are they not both forms of the same thing?

It is a commonplace, is it not, among the medical profession, that each case must be treated individually and differently. The terms "predisposition" and "idiosyncrasy" are applied, in order to justify this difference in treatment. But what, after all, is predisposition and what idiosyncrasy? I am sure that the majority of your professors, when they have the question thus put in a blank, straight-forward manner, would confess practically complete ignorance; but, on the theory of disease expounded by Trall and other hygienic writers, the terms are easily explained. It is merely the greater or lesser encumbrance of the body and blockage of the system with impure material, and the elimination of this material *is* the disease, so-called; the various diseases being merely the various methods of its elimination.

We thus see that all disease has one common cause, and the removal of this cause, - which is in fact the predisposition, - constitutes the 'curing' of the 'disease' . . . .

Then again on the treatment by diet: I read a short time ago Dr. Burney Yeo's lectures on "Food and Diet in Health and Disease", and am glad that I read it - not that I derived any benefit from the book, but because it showed me the hopeless muddle in which the medical world is as present regarding this question of diet! Thus, there is a fundamental principle which seems to be entirely overlooked, and it is this: that because we have digressed amazingly from our natural habits, with regard to food, it proves that these perverted habits are better! No physician would entertain for a moment the idea that impure air is better than pure air, - no matter how long we had been accustomed to the former. He would demand an immediate change to pure air. Yet he is unwilling to grant the same thing with regard to food. If the stomach can be accustomed to unnatural food, because it has subsisted upon it for a long time, does this prove that it cannot become again accustomed to natural food? I see no reason why it should not.

I wish to call your attention to the unifying character of my energy-theory, - apart from its purely practical value. If patients could once realize that, by skipping a meal, they do not lose either bodily heat or strength, but only the amount of tissue which that meal would form; and that, in opposition to this, they have gained the amount of energy that would have been expended in the digestion of that meal, we should have a tremendous revolution in medical methods. . . . . Further, this theory might enable us to explain other strange facts. Take, for instance, the cases of so-called "miraculous healing." Many cases are on record of this kind, which have never been fully explained. Now, on my theory, it is conceivable that, since the vitality of the body is not derived from food, but from some other source - the body being charged with it, so to speak, and the degree of this re-charge being proportional to the condition of the system, - we might conceive that, through a combination of mental, physical and perhaps spiritual causes, the body of the patient might be re-charged more rapidly and effectually than normally, and more powerfully, so that the healing process might go-on far more rapidly than normally, and a "cure" effected in far shorter time. It is theoretically possible, is it not?

All this bears upon the question of sleep - about which so little seems to be known, physiologically. I shall have a long chapter on sleep in my forthcoming book, and shall be interested in hearing what you think of it. It hinges, as you will see, on the vitality theory. . . .

Very sincerely yours,

HEREWARD CARRINGTON.

INDEX

Lightning Source UK Ltd.
Milton Keynes UK
UKOW021558221012

200991UK00010B/78/P